MEDICAL PROCEDURES, TES

A CLOSER LOOK AT AUTOPSIES

FERNANDO ROBERTSON
EDITOR

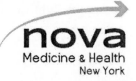

nova
Medicine & Health
New York

Copyright © 2020 by Nova Science Publishers, Inc.

NOTICE TO THE READER

Additional color graphics may be available in the e-book version of this book.

Library of Congress Cataloging-in-Publication Data

ISBN: 978-1-53617-178-5

Published by Nova Science Publishers, Inc. † *New York*

MEDICAL PROCEDURES, TESTING AND TECHNOLOGY

A CLOSER LOOK AT AUTOPSIES

MEDICAL PROCEDURES, TESTING AND TECHNOLOGY

Additional books and e-books in this series can be found on Nova's website under the Series tab.

CONTENTS

PREFACE

From its earliest forerunners in Egyptian mummification and the influence of Herophilus and Galen in ancient Greece, the autopsy has deep roots in the historical effort to understand the human body. Advances in modern post-mortem examination technique, such as non-invasive imaging, will continue to shape the structure and role of the autopsy as it evolves and changes into the future.

The autopsy is a major aspect of the practice of medicine which is used to audit the effectiveness of clinical practice and assist the law courts in the adjudication of cases in which deaths occurred in suspicious circumstances in order to guarantee a safe society, prevent secret homicide, premature deaths and avoid miscarriage of justice.

Practical, legal and ethical aspects of the molecular autopsy method are also discussed. Early diagnosis by genetic testing will force lifestyle modifications in individuals with genetic risk factors, which alone or in combination with other therapeutic options may delay the onset of the disease.

On-site examinations at autopsy in forensic practice are discussed. Since such "on-site" examinations are simple and not time-consuming, the results can be obtained promptly and may be useful for forensic diagnosis.

Autopsy rates have dramatically declined in the last several decades. As such, the authors explore the myriad of aspects that may be contributing to this downward trend.

At a societal level, autopsies play a crucial role in public health and the justice system. They are necessary in understanding the causes and course of epidemic outbreaks and recognizing the emergence of new diseases.

The goal of the concluding chapter is to examine religious beliefs around death and common reasons why religion may be invoked when deciding not to consent to an autopsy. Religions that will be examined include Judaism, Islam, Christianity, Christian Science, Church of Jesus Christ of Latter Day Saints, Jehovah's Witness, Hinduism, and Buddhism.

Chapter 1 - The autopsy in its current form emerged in the 19th century, but its origins started millennia earlier. From its earliest forerunners in Egyptian mummification and the influence of Herophilus and Galen in ancient Greece, the autopsy has deep roots in the historical effort to understand the human body. Developments across the post-classical world, from advances in forensic pathology in Song dynasty China to early European efforts to determine causes of death for individuals, provided a more robust academic framework for the autopsy. Changing religious views on postmortem dissection and the start of the Italian Renaissance led to rapid developments in anatomy and pathology, fueled by human cadaveric dissection. These breakthroughs in pathology were crucial in shaping the development of the autopsy from its role in understanding anatomy to a tool in uncovering the basis of disease into the 17th and 18th centuries;however, it was not until the 19th century when the autopsy could be recognized in its modern incarnation, refined by famed physicians like Karl Rokitansky and Rudolf Virchow. Advances in modern post-mortem examination technique, such as non-invasive imaging, will continue to shape the structure and role of the autopsy as it evolves and changes into the future.

Chapter 2 - The autopsy is a major aspect of the practice of medicine which is used to audit the effectiveness of clinical practice and assist the law courts in the adjudication of cases in which deaths occurred in suspicious circumstances in order to guarantee a safe society, prevent secret homicide, premature deaths and avoid miscarriage of justice. As it happens with all human endeavours, the practice of medicine is a rich and variable blend of science and art and as such it is prone to the influence of human frailties and idiosyncrasies. Many variables affect the conduct, interpretation and conclusion of the autopsy. Thus, guidelines need to be put in place to prevent the pathologist from exploiting the circumstances to an unwholesome advantage of performing below the expected standard of care with regards to the autopsy. No human is under any compulsion to always do the needful except there is the watchtower of the law with untoward consequences and punitive measures for deviants. Therefore it is imperative for the pathologist to know that his practice of autopsy pathology and its derivatives such as clinical and forensic autopsies may be scrutinised by the law courts to ascertain conformity with the standard of care so that his professional opinion does not affect the living through the miscarriage of justice or give a wrong impression as to the cause of death of a deceased person. Such legal scrutiny may be provoked by the decedent's family who may not be pleased by the standard of care at autopsy such as poor presentation of autopsy findings which reflects poor attention to details on the part of the pathologist or outright incompetence. A failure to diagnosis or wrong diagnosis of the cause of death may have a boomeranging effect on the families especially in familial disorders, failure of insurance claims and grievous public health implications for epidemics of infectious diseases. The law therefore continues to keep watch on the specialist in the discipline of anatomical pathology and enables him to maintain appropriate standards in his practice.. Further measures to avoid squabbles with the law and professional hiccups include the pathologist and his supportive staff being absolutely conversant with the jurisdictional requirements of his practice and adhere strictly to such prescriptions except under extenuating circumstances, and even in such situations, anatomical pathologists should make thorough documentation for posterity.

Chapter 3 - In many countries, clinical autopsy rates (i.e., clinical autopsies other than those required by law) have been declining since the 1950s, as a reflection of a clear trend to reduce the importance of the autopsies. This can be attributed to different causes: overreliance on modern diagnostic research techniques, conflicting beliefs and practices regarding treatment of the dead, or fear of lawsuits if results contradict antemortem diagnosis. But autopsy's utility is incontrovertible. The many benefits of autopsy for patients, families, public health and society include identification of factors of interest to family members. For example, in cases in which a fatal lesion may have had an inherited genetic cause, it may be worthwhile to use tissues (taken during autopsy) for molecular DNA analysis. The findings could be used to counsel the family of the deceased about the risks of inherited disease and about the possible prophylactic measures available. Usually, this practice is defined "molecular autopsy." The first author who used the term "molecular autopsy" was Ackerman in 2001, when he performed a molecular autopsy on a 17-year-old boy found dead in bed. By the date, many studies were conducted for molecular identification of susceptibility genes and mutations involved in sudden cardiac death. In this chapter, the authors will discuss practical, legal and ethical aspects of this method. The use of autopsy - expecially of the molecular autopsy - results for medical care, education, research, innovation and health administration provides a good motivation for including autopsy and molecular autopsy as important guarantor of safety of patients and their relatives. The early diagnosis by genetic testing will force lifestyle modifications in individuals (the relatives of the deceased) with genetic risk factors, which alone or in combination with other therapeutic options may delay the onset of the disease. New drugs can also be developed using these genes as targets, which may drive the paradigm shift in modern medicine to personalized medicine.

Chapter 4 - Postmortem biological samples such as blood, urine, bile, tissues, or other materials are collected at forensic autopsy. Various kinds of examinations, including toxicological, microbiological, biochemical, and serological examinations, would be requested from the pathologist. With recent technological developments, some of these examinations can be performed on site, using a single-use device, light portable instruments or examination kits. Since such "on-site" examinations are simple and not time-consuming, the results can be obtained promptly and would be useful for forensic diagnosis.

In the present paper, on-site examinations at autopsy in forensic practice are discussed.

Chapter 5 - The importance of performing autopsies has been recognized for centuries. Despite this, autopsy rates in the last several decades have dramatically fallen off. This chapter explores the myriad aspects that may be contributing to this downward trend. Many clinicians feel uncomfortable requesting autopsies. Many of these same clinicians have never seen an autopsy performed; it is not a requirement of medical school education anymore. Many clinicians operate under the false assumption that with modern technology, autopsies do not add anything and are obsolete. In fact, the rates of missed diagnoses found at autopsy have not changed dramatically, despite these advances in technology. There is also a fear that findings uncovered at autopsy may be used as medicolegal weapons against the physician caregiver. Pathologists who perform autopsies find it a burden, particularly since there is no financial compensation for performing them. Although hospitals pay lip service to autopsies' importance as a quality control measure, they too see autopsies as a money loser.

Chapter 6 - Autopsies have been performed for centuries and historically have served a variety of purposes. In more recent years, autopsy rates have significantly declined and some have argued that the autopsy has become somewhat obsolete given advances in technology and medicine. This article will review the purposes of performing autopsies and their continued relevancy. At a societal level, autopsies play a crucial role in public health and the justice system. They are necessary in understanding the causes and course of epidemic outbreaks and recognizing the emergence of new diseases. In the forensic area, autopsies are performed to explain the cause, mechanism, and manner of death. At an individual level, autopsies allow for a more complete understanding of a patient's disease course which may not have been clear while the patient was alive. This can provide great services to both medical teams and family members of the deceased. Even with advances in medicine, autopsies still uncover missed diagnoses. Much of what we know about many diseases today is the result of autopsies, and in fact, many diseases were first discovered and described at autopsy. Furthermore, autopsies provide a vehicle for ensuring quality care by providing information needed to develop safer medical practices, procedures, and instruments. These examinations can also help families both by bringing closure to the loss of a loved one and potentially uncovering familial or genetic diseases.

Chapter 7 - Although religious beliefs about death and dying are variable, most religions believe autopsies are acceptable if desired by the individual and/or next of kin for special circumstances. Nonetheless, religion is a commonly cited reason for denying autopsy. The goal of this chapter is to examine religious beliefs around death and common reasons why religion may be invoked when deciding not to consent to an autopsy. Religions that will be examined include Judaism, Islam, Christianity (Catholicism and Protestantism), Christian Science, Church of Jesus Christ of Latter Day Saints (Mormon), Jehovah's Witness, Hinduism, and Buddhism.

In: A Closer Look at Autopsies
Editor: Fernando Robertson
ISBN: 978-1-53617-178-5
© 2020 Nova Science Publishers, Inc.

Chapter 1

THE HISTORY OF THE AUTOPSY: FROM ANCIENT EGYPT INTO THE FUTURE

*David D. Xiong[1], Julie Y. Zhou[2] and Richard A. Prayson[1,3,]**

[1]Cleveland Clinic Lerner College of Medicine,
Cleveland Clinic, Cleveland, OH, US
[2]Department of Pathology,
Case Western Reserve University School of Medicine,
Cleveland, OH, US
[3]Department of Anatomic Pathology, Cleveland Clinic,
Cleveland, OH, US

ABSTRACT

The autopsy in its current form emerged in the 19th century, but its origins started millennia earlier. From its earliest forerunners in Egyptian mummification and the influence of Herophilus and Galen in ancient Greece, the autopsy has deep roots in the historical effort to understand the human body. Developments across the post-classical world, from

[*] Corresponding author: Richard Prayson, MD, MEd, Department of Anatomic Pathology, L25, Cleveland Clinic, 9500 Euclid Avenue, Cleveland, OH 44195 USA, Phone: 216-444-8805, FAX: 216-445-6967, E-mail: praysor@ccf.,org.

advances in forensic pathology in Song dynasty China to early European efforts to determine causes of death for individuals, provided a more robust academic framework for the autopsy. Changing religious views on postmortem dissection and the start of the Italian Renaissance led to rapid developments in anatomy and pathology, fueled by human cadaveric dissection. These breakthroughs in pathology were crucial in shaping the development of the autopsy from its role in understanding anatomy to a tool in uncovering the basis of disease into the 17th and 18th centuries;however, it was not until the 19th century when the autopsy could be recognized in its modern incarnation, refined by famed physicians like Karl Rokitansky and Rudolf Virchow. Advances in modern post-mortem examination technique, such as non-invasive imaging, will continue to shape the structure and role of the autopsy as it evolves and changes into the future.

INTRODUCTION

The modern autopsy is a systematic examination of the gross and microscopic details of the human body for gaining an understanding of its processes during life and contributors to its death. Its gradual evolution into its current state winds through much of medicine's recorded history. In addition, the development of the autopsy is intimately tied to progress in the field of human anatomy because the inspection of internal organs is essential to the foundational knowledge base that the modern autopsy requires.

ANCIENT EGYPT

The earliest recorded roots of autopsy and the study of human anatomy originated from the practices of mummification in ancient Egypt. These methods only crudely resemble the modern autopsy. Embalmers prepared bodies by removing internal organs and placing them in four Canopic jars that were thought to preserve the organs needed for the afterlife. Despite the invasive nature of mummification and its similarity in appearance to the autopsy, there was no known application of the knowledge obtained from mummification to the practice of medicine or pathology, as the individuals preparing mummies were not physicians, but instead embalmers, who were of a lower social caste (J. L. Burton 2005; King and Meehan 1973). In addition, documentation of the technical aspects of mummification from ancient Egypt was scarce. The vast majority of ancient documents detailing the mummification process are concerned with the religious ceremonies, incantations, and funerary rites of the deceased (King and Meehan 1973; J. L. Burton 2005). Only two surviving papyri from ancient Egypt make any note of the actual process of mummification and embalming, and neither remark on anatomic or medical considerations. The *Papyrus of the Embalming Ritual*, for example, is an incomplete first century CE document recording the process of cleaning and preparing the body for mummification that does not document any examination or study of the body, its internal organs, or disease processes that the deceased may have suffered from (Riggs 2010). Thus, though the Egyptians must have made observations regarding anatomy and pathology from the deceased, there are no indications that this information was propagated (J. L. Burton 2005; King and Meehan 1973).

There are other scant ancient Egyptian papyri that document anatomic and medical findings in patients, but only one, the *Edwin Smith papyrus*, is notable for largely averting magical or religious influences and instead relies on objective observations (King and Meehan 1973). The *Edwin Smith papyrus* is a text from approximately 1600 BCE documenting 40-some cases of traumatic injuries. These cases, which are almost all traumatic injuries, are organized by their presenting features, the physician's assessment of the injury, and whether treatment was deemed possible (van Middendorp, Sanchez, and Burridge 2010; Hajar 2012a). Since the papyrus was primarily a text for injuries with concrete physical presentations, its significance lies in correlating anatomic injuries to their resulting deficits. Remarkably, the text provides accurate anatomic descriptions of cranial structures including the meninges, brain, and cerebrospinal fluid. Though there are no direct mentions of postmortem examination, discussions of human anatomy, or in-depth discussion of pathology, it represents one of the earliest medical texts tying together anatomy, clinical history, and causes of death (Breasted 1991; Hajar 2012a; van Middendorp, Sanchez, and Burridge 2010).

The *Edwin Smith papyrus* represents an unusual perspective toward medicine and pathology in the ancient world. Spirituality and mysticism permeated much of the understanding of disease and death during this time, including ancient Egyptian and Mesopotamian civilizations (King and Meehan 1973). In these societies, investigation of physical causes of disease and death was often times deemed unnecessary—why open the body when religion and magic already provided adequate explanation? Practices such as haruspicy, the sacrifice of animals and examining the morphology of their liver or digestive organs to interpret the will of the gods, were not uncommon (J. L. Burton 2005; King and Meehan 1973).

THE HELLENISTIC PERIOD AND THE ROMAN EMPIRE

Despite these magical or religious foundations, investigations into the causes of disease continued. The ancient Greeks were instrumental in advancing the notion that disease was caused by natural processes. If these disease processes were found in nature, then they could be investigated by human means, setting the stage for further advances in anatomy and pathology (King and Meehan 1973).

The first well-documented bodies of work on anatomic dissection date from the 3rd century BCE and were written by the Greek physician Herophilus (King and Meehan 1973; J. L. Burton 2005). Herophilus (~335-255 BCE), now credited as the "Father of Anatomy," and his contemporary, Erasistratus (~304-250 BCE), pioneered the study of human anatomy. Both lived and worked in Alexandria, a leading city of intellectualism, learning, and scientific discovery in the Hellenistic period, where for the first time in recorded history, human dissection for academic study was permitted (Ghosh 2015). This progressive environment provided fertile ground for Herophilus to make numerous advances in anatomic knowledge as the first known individual to perform systematic human dissections. His advances include differentiating the gross structure of blood vessels, tendons, and nerves, discovering and naming the duodenum and prostate, and describing the structures of the liver, pancreas, reproductive organs, components of the eye, and the torcular herophili (now more commonly referred to as the confluence of sinuses), a vascular structure in the brain which bears his name (Ghosh 2015; Hajar 2012a; Bay and Bay 2010). Additionally, he theorized that the brain, rather than the heart, was the master organ that controlled the rest of the body (Hajar 2012a; Bay and Bay 2010; Ghosh 2015)

Erasistratus, his younger contemporary, also made significant contributions to anatomy, but he was more interested in its application to physiology. He distinguished between the systemic and pulmonary circulation and hypothesized that the lungs distributed air to the blood, which was then pumped via the heart and arteries to the body, ultimately returning via the veins (Aird 2011). Unfortunately, Herophilus and Erasistratus are among the only known Greek anatomists who engaged in the practice of human dissection, which seems to have fallen out of favor after their deaths. This decline may have been hastened by the growth of a rival school of medical theory which argued that human dissection did not contribute useful knowledge to medicine and effective treatment could only be guided by non-invasive observations (Ghosh 2015). In any case, the practice of human dissection gradually faded from Alexandria. The full works of these two great Greek anatomists were ultimately lost to history by the 3rd or 4th century CE. Our lasting knowledge of their contributions is derived second-hand, primarily from the treatises of Galen, who mentioned many of their discoveries in his own works (Ghosh 2015)

Galen of Pergamon (129-~216 CE) was perhaps the most prominent figure in Greco-Roman medicine, and his work would come to define Western and Islamic medicine for more than a millennium. He spent time training in medicine in Alexandria, and as a physician, treated multitudes of patients including the Roman emperors Marcus Aurelius and Commodus (West 2014). Galen was revered both during and after his life, and his immense stature in academia solidified his ideas for generations. Galen wrote on a wide variety of medical subjects including anatomy and pathology and is believed to have authored a total of 500 to 600 books and treatises, of which only a third survive (van den Tweel and Taylor 2010).

Galen made numerous contributions to anatomy, such as his descriptions of the individual muscles and bones in the body, the structure and function of some of the cranial nerves, and the flow of blood through the vascular system (West 2014). His anatomic work, however, was only based on his dissections of animals, and any possible experience with human anatomy is thought to have been obtained early in his career while examining and treating injured gladiators in his home city (J. L. Burton 2005; West 2014). Some sources suggest that human dissection was outlawed in the Roman empire (Ghosh 2015), but regardless of the cause, Galen never performed a posthumous human dissection. Thus, numerous errors in his descriptions of body parts exist, including incorrect descriptions of the musculature in the hands, the skeletal anatomy of the jaw, sternum, and coccyx, and cardiopulmonary circulation (Savage-Smith 2013; West 2014). His authority in anatomy would not be seriously challenged until Andreas Vesalius' work in the 16th century.

Additionally, Galen's work in pathology and the development of disease was based on the theory of humorism, which is the idea that the body contains four basic fluids (blood, black bile, yellow bile, and phlegm) (West 2014). Balanced proportions of each fluid kept an individual healthy but caused disease and distemperment when balance was disrupted. Hippocrates (~460-370 BCE) first popularized the theory of humorism, but Galen cemented its role as the dominant scientific theory at the time in how diseases originated, and it held significant sway in medicine well into the 17th century (West 2014; Hajar 2012b).

Advancements in anatomy and pathology beyond the time of Galen essentially came to a standstill with the decline of the Roman empire, and no substantial breakthroughs would come from Europe until the 14th century (Ghosh 2015).

NON-EUROPEAN DEVELOPMENTS IN ANATOMY AND THE AUTOPSY

Anatomy and pathology outside of the Western world continued to develop despite the dearth of documented advances in Europe during the dark ages and medieval times. Although many records were lost with the decline and fall of the Roman Empire, the knowledge that the Greek anatomists had built survived. Galen's works were translated into Arabic and disseminated through the Islamic caliphates, where Arabic physicians built on his works and made advances in anatomy and physiology (Alghamdi, Ziermann, and Diogo 2017; Hajar 2013). Arab physicians made many corrections to Galen's work. Prominent examples include advances in understanding blood flow through the heart and pulmonary circulation and refuting the Galenic idea that blood exiting the right ventricle directly enters the left ventricle (Alghamdi, Ziermann, and Diogo 2017). Notable Islamic physicians who contributed to the understanding of human anatomy during this era include Al-Razi (Razes, 865-925), who published several medical encyclopedias; Ibn Sina (Avicenna, 980-1037), who described in detail the organ systems of the body and wrote arguably the single best and most comprehensive medical text (*The Canon of Medicine*) until the 15th century; and Al-Baghdadi (1162-1231), who identified and corrected important errors in Galen's work, such as the anatomy of the mandible, sacrum, and coccyx (Alghamdi, Ziermann, and Diogo 2017). However, it is unclear if this information was based on the dissection of human cadavers or solely through detailed clinical examination and surgery. Human dissection was not particularly in vogue in the Islamic empire, though it was not explicitly prohibited (Savage-Smith 2013; Alghamdi, Ziermann, and Diogo 2017). Islamic medicine began to decline after the Crusades, and much of the knowledge of anatomy and pathology carried through Islamic manuscripts was ultimately translated and spread across Europe at the beginning of the Renaissance (van den Tweel and Taylor 2010; Hajar 2013).

Looking further eastward, ancient India and China also made significant advances in anatomy and pathology. Centuries before the

Common Era, the Sushruta Samhita outlined procedures for the conduct of post-mortem inspection of human bodies, and encouraged the study and dissection of cadavers by students of medicine in order to learn about the body and practice procedures. Interestingly, the Sushruta Samhita also describes a number of relatively advanced plastic surgery procedures, including rhinoplasty and reconstructive flaps (Hajar 2012a; Menon and Haberman 1969). The Charaka Samhita, another ancient Indian medical text, described portions of human anatomy, including bones, muscles, joints, blood vessels, and the heart in the first century CE (Hajar 2012a; Menon and Haberman 1969).

Cultural norms in Ancient China prior to the Yuan Dynasty (1200s) disfavored the dissection of human bodies and thus led to a dearth of anatomic knowledge (Hajar 2012a). However, the Yuan Dynasty was notable for the publication of the first systematic treatise on forensic science, the *Washing Away of Wrongs*. This text was written in the 13th century by Song Ci, a Chinese physician and judge, to help guide government officials in their examination of crime. The work covered the methodology of post-mortem examinations and the determination of a cause of death. This was a seminal work in Chinese medicolegal policy, and was used and revised well into the Ming and Qing dynasties, centuries after its initial publication (Hajar 2012a; Wu 2015).

MIDDLE AGES (400-1200S)

Religious norms in medieval Europe precluded the dissection of human cadavers for more than a millennium and thus substantive advances in anatomy, pathology, and autopsy were lacking. During this time, the dissection of cadavers was considered blasphemous and was generally prohibited in Europe (Ghosh 2015; van den Tweel and Taylor 2013). In addition, overall attitudes toward medicine took a decidedly religious turn after the fall of the Roman Empire. Disease and death were seen as acts of God, and thus human interventions were against divine will - only prayer and faith could cure disease (J. L. Burton 2005).

Despite these attitudes in Europe, the propagation of medical knowledge from surviving Greek and Roman texts continued in the Islamic empire. Human dissections and autopsies were rare in this period, as was the contribution of new knowledge to the fields of anatomy and pathology. Isolated mentions of anatomic dissections or post-mortem examinations are found starting in the 12th century in European accounts. For example, one anecdote recorded in the 12th-century book *Gesta Regum Anglorum* ("Deeds of the Kings of the English") described a primitive autopsy order by Sigurd I Magnusson, King of Norway in 1111 (van den Tweel and Taylor 2013; de Campos and Rocha 2015). While returning from a Crusade, a number of his soldiers died in Constantinople. Suspecting that the deaths had been caused by bad wine, the King ordered a pig's liver to be thrown into the wine, and it became damaged. Then, he ordered one of the dead soldier's bodies opened up to study the liver, and found that it was similarly damaged (King and Meehan 1973; van den Tweel and Taylor 2013; de Campos and Rocha 2015).

However, there appears to be no further systematic development in post-mortem examinations or medical knowledge derived from these events. Multiple changes, however, led to a gradual thaw in the attitudes toward human dissection and a corresponding increase in medical knowledge. Pope Innocent III recommended in 1209 that unexplained deaths should be investigated by a physician, softening religious attitudes toward postmortem investigation as a desecration of a corpse (de Campos and Rocha 2015; van den Tweel and Taylor 2013). In 1231, the Holy Roman Emperor Frederick II (1194-1250) decreed that a human body should be dissected every five years in his empire, and students of medicine and surgery were required to be in attendance (Ghosh 2015). Later, a decree issued by Pope Nicholas IV in 1292 permitted graduates of the medical school of the University of Bologna to teach anatomy worldwide, bolstering the popularity and reputation of the university and attracting students from many countries to study at Bologna (Ghosh 2015). Matching these changes, recorded postmortem examinations to determine causes of death started in Italy in the late 1200s as well (J. L. Burton 2005; King and Meehan 1973; Ghosh 2015). All of these factors combined to create the fertile climate for the resurgence of anatomy in the coming years.

Nevertheless, advances in human dissection only came haltingly. In 1299, Pope Boniface VIII issued a decree, *De Sepulturis*, which prohibited the separation of flesh from the bones of the dead. This was aimed at stopping the trafficking of human remains of soldiers who had died in Crusades or wars abroad. This decree may have been interpreted in varying degrees as prohibiting the dissection of human bodies and autopsy (J. L. Burton 2005; King and Meehan 1973; Ghosh 2015; Gulczyński, Iżycka-Świeszewska, and Grzybiak 2009).

END OF THE MIDDLE AGES, BEGINNING OF THE RENAISSANCE (1300s)

The autopsy as a dedicated technique for medical examination started taking root in the Renaissance era. Despite the fervent atmosphere of intellectualism and dissemination of medical knowledge at the University of Bologna, academic human dissections only resumed at the institution in 1315 after a hiatus of over a millennium (Ghosh 2015). Mondino de Luzzi, a prominent Italian physician and anatomist, performed this first dissection and subsequent dissections were performed at least annually at the university. These dissections were multi-day events where the bodies of multiple executed criminals were opened for the purpose of teaching anatomy (Ghosh 2015).

However, the academic value of these early dissections is unclear due to the manner in which anatomy was taught at the time. Human dissections were presided over by a team of instructors. The professor of anatomy (*lector*, lecturer) would read from an anatomy text (usually one of Galen's texts) and oversee the dissection, while the professor's assistant (*ostensor*) would point at the structure being described in the text. Finally, the lowly barber-surgeon (*sector*) was the only individual who actually touched and dissected the cadaver for students to observe (Zampieri et al. 2015). Due to this separation in roles, the physical separation between the professor and the cadaver, the perceived 'infallibility' of Galen and the anatomic texts, and the relegation of the actual human body as a mere conduit to learn from the text, there was little growth in the body of anatomic knowledge during this time (Ghosh 2015; Barr 2015).

Nevertheless, this increase in dissections was important for setting the stage for further advances in anatomy and pathology. As governmental and religious views relaxed on human dissection and postmortem examination, societal attitudes toward dissection softened as well, and human dissection spread throughout Italian medical schools (Ghosh 2015).

Postmortem autopsies to determine disease course and causes of death became more commonly documented as well, with examples of autopsies conducted for medicolegal inquiries into causes of death. The black death, which ravaged Europe in the mid-1300s, provided multiple instances where wealthy aristocrats and leaders financed postmortem examinations in order to investigate the victims' cause of death (J. L. Burton 2005; Ghosh 2015).

FIFTEENTH CENTURY (1400S)

By the 15th century, autopsies began to include prominent individuals. When Antipope Alexander V died suddenly in 1410, poisoning was suspected, and an autopsy was performed to identify a cause of death though the results were unclear (King and Meehan 1973; Gulczyński, Iżycka-Świeszewska, and Grzybiak 2009). Volumes of clinical reports and autopsies were published and circulated as well. One of the prime examples is the book *De abditis nonnullis ac mirandis morborum et sanationum causis* (*On some remarkable hidden causes of disease and healing*), a compendium of cases published by the renowned Florentine physician Antonio Benivieni (J. L. Burton 2005; King and Meehan 1973; van den Tweel and Taylor 2013). This book was a collection of 111 of his cases, of which about 15 included autopsy reports to further investigate the cause of death. At this point, however, autopsy reports were in their infancy. Only a brief statement or sentence of the most important findings was provided, and no other observations or organs were remarked upon. For example, Benivieni describes the case of a man who vomited almost all of his food and died from malnourishment. The entirety of the autopsy report is as follows: "It was found that the opening of his stomach had closed up and it had hardened down to the lowest part with the result that nothing could pass through to the organs beyond, and death inevitably followed" (King and Meehan 1973). Another case describes a woman who had suffered from chronic abdominal pain and painful and infrequent bowel movements, and upon her death her autopsy showed a thick callus compressing her intestines, leaving only a narrow channel for stool. This was the only finding recorded in the autopsy report (King and Meehan 1973). Nevertheless, autopsies had become so commonplace that it was unusual enough for Benivieni to note when a family refused an autopsy of a deceased individual (J. L. Burton 2005; King and Meehan 1973).

Similar tomes, such as Giovanni Rosati's *De abditis morborum causis*, ("*The hidden causes of disease*") were published by Bienvieni's contemporaries and represented some of the first books on anatomic pathology (Gulczyński, Iżycka-Świeszewska, and Grzybiak 2009). In addition to the growth in information, religious attitudes toward autopsies continued changing as well. Pope Sixtus IV, in the late 1400s, permitted the dissection of the human body, which was subsequently confirmed by Pope Clement VII (J. L. Burton 2005).

SIXTEENTH CENTURY (1500S)

Though autopsies were increasingly commonplace, knowledge of human anatomy had not changed significantly since the time of Galen. Many physicians and anatomists held strongly to Galenic views of medicine, much in the same way as today's clinicians reference modern anatomy texts like *Gray's Anatomy*, and were thus not seeking to question or overturn conventional thought in anatomy or pathology (Ghosh 2015). More so, professors and clinicians were loath to do the dissections themselves but rather relied on the lower social class *sectors* to perform the actual dissections while they, their students, and assistants observed (Barr 2015; Zampieri et al. 2015). Thus, opportunities to substantively challenge Galen's dogma were sparse despite the increases in recorded autopsies.

This would all change with the work of Andreas Vesalius. Vesalius was born in Brussels in 1514, and was a figure so important to the history of anatomy that it is sometimes divided into pre-Vesalius and post-Vesalius eras (Hadzic et al. 2014). He started his career as a promising young student, was appointed as the Chair of the Department of Surgery at the University of Padua the day after he graduated from that same university in 1538, and quickly ascended to prominence as an anatomist (Barr 2015). Vesalius made many important contributions to the foundation of anatomy and is credited as one of the most important figures in transforming anatomy and the autopsy (Zampieri et al. 2015).

Vesalius was especially instrumental in questioning the infallibility of Galen and his ideas, which had influenced western medicine for more than a millennium. As a professor, Vesalius taught anatomy through dissection and personally performed many autopsies. He was a revolutionary anatomist and worked as the *lector*, *ostentor*, and *sector* in his dissections, three previously separate roles. In doing so, he emphasized that one must not rely on gaining anatomic knowledge from the ancient texts, but rather gathered from the cadaver directly in front of them (Zampieri et al. 2015). By performing human dissections, he discovered and publicized hundreds of errors in Galen's works. In doing so, Vesalius inferred that Galen's anatomic findings were based on animal dissections and not human dissections (Gulczyński, Iżycka-Świeszewska, and Grzybiak 2009, 2011). His opus magnum, *De human corporis fabrica septem libri* (*Seven books on the fabric of the human body*) was published in 1543 and consolidated his findings into one massive work consisting of 663 pages and 420 illustrations (Barr 2015; Zampieri et al. 2015). These illustrations were especially noteworthy not only for their high quality but also because the majority of prior anatomy textbooks relied on verbal descriptions instead of pictures to describe human anatomy (Barr 2015). He published an updated version of the work in 1555 which extolled even more forcefully the need for anatomic studies of human cadavers and cautioned against blind reliance on anatomic texts (Zampieri et al. 2015).

In addition to his academic work, Vesalius was employed as a physician and surgeon to the Holy Roman Emperor Charles V and made use of his extensive knowledge of anatomy (Barr 2015). He, along with others, attempted to save King Henry II of France after he was mortally injured in a jousting tournament by a fragment of a lance entering his orbit. After the ultimately unsuccessful attempt, Vesalius autopsied the king and prepared his autopsy report, connecting the clinical history of the orbital injury with the autopsy findings (Zampieri et al. 2015). Aristocrats and nobles likewise would request autopsies for their family members upon their death (J. L. Burton 2005; Zampieri et al. 2015).

As the practice of autopsies spread, increasing insight into disease processes gathered as well. Pieter Pauw (1564-1617) provides an exemplary case in one of his autopsy reports. Pauw performed an autopsy on the young daughter of a prominent Dutch individual who had suffered from a history of blindness and thirst. Upon entering the skull, Pauw noted that he "found a significant vesicle, that had occupied the optic nerves close to their crossing, and when I cut it open half a pound of the clearest of watery material flowed out" (J. L. Burton 2005). This is the first known report of an arachnoid cyst causing diabetes insipidus.

SEVENTEENTH CENTURY (1600s)

Human dissections increased in frequency into the 17th century, but not necessarily for altruistic reasons. Since common Christian belief at the time was that a preserved body was necessary for the resurrection and afterlife, dissections of executed criminals became more common as an additional punishment that would destroy their body and prevent them from reaching heaven (J. L. Burton 2005). These practices were documented in two well-known paintings by Rembrandt van Rijn, *The Anatomy Lesson of Dr. Nicolaes Tulp*, and *The Anatomy Lesson of Dr. Joan Deyman* (J. L. Burton 2005; Ghosh 2015). *The Anatomy Lesson of*

Dr. Nicolaes Tulp, the more recognized painting, depicted Dr. Tulp, who was at that time the mayor of Amsterdam as well as a respected physician and anatomist, dissecting the arm of an executed criminal and explaining the anatomy to an audience of onlookers in 1632 (Ghosh 2015; J. L. Burton 2005; Gulczyński, Iżycka-Świeszewska, and Grzybiak 2011). This is an intriguing snapshot into societal attitudes toward dissection, as it indicates that dissections had now moved fully into the public sphere and even became somewhat of a social event. Through the late 1500s and 1600s, autopsy theatres were built across Europe to house audiences for anatomic dissections and anyone who could pay an entrance fee (physicians, students, and the general public) could enter and watch as the anatomist performed a dissection (J. L. Burton 2005).

The prevalence of autopsies increased as well during the 1600s. In 1613, the first fetal autopsy in Northern and Central Europe was performed and published (Gulczyński, Iżycka-Świeszewska, and Grzybiak 2011) and in 1661, the first recorded autopsy was performed in the United States (C 1978). The autopsies of prominent individuals started being publicized, including King Henry IV (1610), King James I (1625), Prince Henry (the Prince of Wales, 1612), John Pym (leader of the English parliament, 1643) and Thomas "Old" Parr (who was allegedly 152 years old at his death, 1635) (J. L. Burton 2005). Interestingly, the concerns regarding the integrity of the body and its ability to enter the afterlife after an autopsy were not as grave compared to a postmortem anatomic dissection. The skeleton was considered to be the key component of an individual's body, and an autopsy would not have separated or damaged the bones as much as a more thorough and systematic dissection (J. L. Burton 2005). In addition, prominent or unusual deaths, such as in the cases of John Pym, Elisabetta Sirani, and Princess Henrietta-Ann of England, were widely published and discussed in public, further increasing public awareness, familiarity, and acceptance of the autopsy (J. L. Burton 2005).

Concordant with the increase in autopsies, numerous physicians began publishing books of their autopsy findings. Theophile Bonet (1620-1689) authored perhaps the most noteworthy compilation of autopsy reports, as his book, *Sepulchretum sive anatomia practica ex cadaveribis morbo denatis* (*Repository of anatomical studies practiced on corpses affected by disease*), assembled 3,000 autopsy reports in two 1,700 page volumes (King and Meehan 1973; van den Tweel and Taylor 2013). These cases included not only Bonet's own autopsies but also included cases collected and published from the last 2 centuries (King and Meehan 1973; van den Tweel and Taylor 2010; de Campos and Rocha 2015).

William Harvey (1578-1657) was another very influential physician who contributed significantly to the fields of anatomy and pathology during the 17th century. He is best known for being the first to describe completely, and in detail, the correct flow of blood through the circulatory system and the central role of the heart in circulation in his book *Exercitatio anatomica de motucordis et sanguinis in animalibus* (*An anatomic exercise on the motion of the heart and blood in living beings*, 1628) (West 2014). In addition, he further developed the ability of the autopsy to investigate disease by tying together multiple autopsy findings in an individual to a single disease process, noting that a patient with aortic valve insufficiency also had left ventricular hypertrophy and ventricular rupture (van den Tweel and Taylor 2010; West 2014).

EIGHTEENTH CENTURY (1700S)

As autopsy reports continued to be published and discussed, Herman Boerhaave (1668-1738) emphasized the need for a complete examination of the body, lest some inconspicuous or seemingly unimportant detail critical to the case be overlooked (J. L. Burton 2005). In addition, he emphasized the importance of clinicopathologic correlation in determining the cause of death, and published many autopsy cases that discussed and related a patient's clinical history to their autopsy findings (van den Tweel and Taylor 2010). As a testament to his attention to detail, Boerhaave reported the autopsy findings of the Dutch Admiral Baron Jan van Wassenaer, who had ingested a rather large meal, vomited, and died soon after in 1724. His autopsy report spanned a full six pages, describing the fatal esophageal rupture and the rest of the autopsy findings at length. This phenomenon—esophageal rupture caused by forceful vomiting—is today named Boerhaave syndrome (J. L. Burton 2005; van den Tweel and Taylor 2013).

Another important 18th century anatomist, Giovanni Battista Morgagni (1682-1771) was one of the champions of the modern autopsy. Like Boerhaave, he emphasized the need to understand the relationship between a patient's clinical history and the findings at autopsy (van den Tweel and Taylor 2013; de Campos and Rocha 2015). He placed considerable emphasis on the use of the autopsy as a tool to understand disease and pondered the medical progress that could have been made if autopsies had been more widely accepted earlier (J. L. Burton 2005). His opus magnum, *De Sedibus et Causis Morborum per Anotomen Indagatis* (*On the seats and causes of diseases, investigated by anatomy*), included 640 autopsies and correlated the anatomic findings with the history of disease in these cases (J. L. Burton 2005; van den Tweel and Taylor 2010; de Campos and Rocha 2015).

Morgani died in 1771, the same year that Xavier Bichat (1771-1802), the "Father of Modern Histology," was born. Bichat further defined the autopsy by focusing not only on the organs but also on the different tissues that composed the bodily organs and characterized their properties (de Campos and Rocha 2015; van den Tweel and Taylor 2013). Remarkably, this was accomplished without the help of a microscope, but rather with simple methods such as cooking, boiling, freezing, putrefaction, and other physical and chemical procedures (van den Tweel and Taylor 2013). Bichat viewed the autopsy as integral to the practice of the physician, in order to achieve a more complete understanding of the body and disease (J. L. Burton 2005; King and Meehan 1973).

NINETEENTH CENTURY (1800S)

The 19th century saw a rise in the practice of autopsies that coincided with advances in science and the technology. Rapid development of scientific fields such as chemistry and physiology guided the development of a more scientific approach to the study of pathology, and technologic advances gave the pathologist more tools to interrogate the questions at hand. Chief among these tools was the popularization of the light microscope in pathology. While microscopy had been used since the late 17th century in biology, it was not widely used in anatomy, pathology, or autopsies until the 19th century (van den Tweel and Taylor 2010; King and Meehan 1973; Gulczyński, Iżycka-Świeszewska, and Grzybiak 2011). This transition between gross and microscopic examination can be exemplified in the two most influential pathologists of the century: Karl Rokitansky (1804-1878) and Rudolf Virchow (1821-1902).

Rokitansky was a master of the autopsy as a gross examination. He was renowned for conducting more than 30,000 autopsies while supervising another 70,000 during career (Stenn 1971; J. L. Burton 2005), and is considered the father of the modern-day autopsy and credited with developing pathology into an independent field (van den Tweel and Taylor 2013). He developed the concept for a standardized systematic autopsy with the full examination of each organ (J. L. Burton 2005; van den Tweel and Taylor 2013) and published a remarkable text, *Handbuch der pathologischen Anatomie* (*A manual of pathological anatomy*), which documented many of his autopsy findings and set standards of work for pathologists (Gulczyński, Iżycka-Świeszewska, and Grzybiak 2011). Rokitansky's focus was on understanding the disease through a unification of clinical and pathologic findings, tracing the development of disease and correlating autopsy findings and clinical history along the way. However, for better or for worse, he purposefully separated his work as a pathologist from his role as a clinician, and often did not take into account the clinical history prior to performing the autopsy. This was done to minimize bias in the autopsy, as many physicians only paid attention to the organs which they *a priori* believed to be the cause of disease, but it marked the beginning of the separation between pathology and clinical medicine (J. L. Burton 2005; Gulczyński, Iżycka-Świeszewska, and Grzybiak 2011).

Rokitansky infrequently made use of the microscope in pathologic examination and thus, sometimes constructed hypotheses that were incongruent with contemporary academic knowledge. For example, he believed that diseases resulted from abnormalities in the blood, and these diseases in turn caused even more abnormalities in the blood, leading to a self-propagating cycle of disease (van den Tweel and Taylor 2010). Because Rokitansky believed that blood abnormalities caused disease, he also believed that chemical analysis of the blood would be key in pursuing a greater understanding of pathology. Rudolf Virchow rightly criticized this view as resembling humorism and "a monstrous anachronism," and it was subsequently omitted from Rokitansky's publications in the future (van den Tweel and Taylor 2010).

Virchow, who once trained under Rokitansky, built upon the work that Rokitansky had established and made great contributions to the modern understanding of pathology with extensive use of the microscope, advancing the knowledge of pathology to a cellular level (J. L. Burton 2005). The existence of cells and the fact that they were the building blocks of animal life was already known, but Virchow was instrumental in recognizing the ability of cells to self-replicate (the third tenet of cell theory) and famously uttered: "Omnis cellula e cellula" ("From cells come cells") (van den Tweel and Taylor 2010). This change in dogma provoked an immense shift in pathology, especially with the widespread publication of his book espousing cellular theory in 1859, *Die Cellularpathologie* (*Cellular Pathology*) (van den Tweel and Taylor 2010). No longer was the whole body, individual organs, or tissue the smallest unit of the body affected by disease, but rather the body's cells. Thus, cells had to be examined to find the causes of disease, and cellular changes rather than a constellation of symptoms could be used to classify and investigate disease, leading to much clearer classifications of disease and significantly improving diagnostic and prognostic accuracy (van den Tweel and Taylor 2010). This led to the growth of the field of histopathology, using the microscope to unravel further the cellular basis of disease and death. There was an explosion in developments, with new techniques for staining and examining tissue like paraffin embedding, formaldehyde fixation, and hematoxylin and eosin staining (van den Tweel and Taylor 2010; de Campos and Rocha 2015).

In addition to Virchow's work in cellular pathology, he also published a small book detailing the procedures and practice of the autopsies that he conducted (van den Tweel and Taylor 2013). He again echoed the refrain that all organs must be thoroughly examined, and that a properly conducted autopsy would thus last at least three hours (de Campos and Rocha 2015). In his autopsies, he removed each organ one by one and examined them separately. For his work in developing cellular pathology, he is considered by some as the greatest individual in the history of pathology (J. L. Burton 2005).

Sir William Osler (1849-1919), another revered physician in modern medicine, is said to have performed approximately a thousand autopsies himself, wrote a five-volume work on autopsy procedure, and depended on autopsy findings to hone his clinical craft (J. L. Burton 2005).

TWENTIETH CENTURY (1900s) HEIGHTS AND THE AUTOPSY'S MODERN DECLINE

Given the relative paucity of diagnostic techniques as definitive as the autopsy, it stood to reason that much of medical knowledge prior to modern laboratory testing was derived from autopsy findings. This was further reinforced in various ways during the 20th century. Richard Cabot, a physician working in the early 20th century, started the clinicopathologic conference in order to further strengthen the connection between the understanding of clinical history and pathologic findings during autopsy (C. S. Roberts 1990). In 1912, he published a controversial yet influential paper documenting significant discrepancies between the clinically determined cause of death and the pathologic cause of death identified at autopsy (Cabot 1912). This was a finding which strengthened the necessity of the autopsy as a tool to ensure quality control for clinical diagnosis as well as a learning tool in order to improve future diagnoses (C. S. Roberts 1990). Between Cabot's work and other contemporary influences in medical education, such as the release of the Flexner Report in 1910, the groundwork was set for an increase in autopsies in the United States (King and Meehan 1973). Indeed, until the advent of biomedical and clinical research as a major driving factor in academic reputation later in the 20th century, the autopsy rate often times played a major role in a hospital's reputation (King and Meehan 1973).

The 19th and 20th centuries saw the heyday of autopsies, but various factors acted to gradually curtail the prevalence of autopsies. Perhaps chief among them was the increasing development of clinical testing, such as laboratory and chemistry testing, and radiographic studies. This served to put increasing emphasis on diagnostic testing of the living, a change that gradually shifted value and financial incentives away from the autopsy toward clinical pathology (King and Meehan 1973; van den Tweel and Taylor 2013). With the removal of reimbursement for autopsies from the Centers of Medicare and Medicaid and the removal of the requirement for autopsies for hospital accreditation by the Joint Commission, among other factors, there were no longer major reasons for hospital systems to pursue autopsies, and not as much incentive to persuade patients and families to conduct them (Shojania and Burton 2008). As a result, elective autopsy rates have been gradually declining since the mid-20th century (Shojania and Burton 2008). Though a significant minority (~20%) of all deaths entail a medicolegal autopsy, less than 10% of all deaths are currently followed by an autopsy in the United States (Hoyert, DL 2011; Shojania and Burton 2008).

Postmortem examination techniques have continued evolving to encompass minimally invasive examination techniques in order to supplement or even serve as an alternative to a conventional autopsy, especially for families hesitant to give permission for an invasive autopsy. Postmortem computed tomography (CT) and magnetic resonance imaging (MRI) examinations, angiography, and image-guided tissue biopsies can give anatomic information and even minimally invasive tissue samples for histopathologic testing (Okuda et al. 2013). Research is currently being conducted on incorporating and refining this technique for postmortem examination. For example, Japan has a significantly lower autopsy rate than similarly developed Western countries and thus, has more fully implemented the use of postmortem imaging as a replacement for the autopsy as well as to identify cases that may benefit from an autopsy (Okuda et al. 2013). However, current postmortem imaging examination techniques still have significant shortcomings. CT cannot detect direct evidence of some common causes of death like acute heart failure, and MRI has significantly reduced availability and is much more time-consuming than CT (Okuda et al. 2013). Additionally, errors rates in both postmortem CT and MRI still preclude its widespread use as a replacement for autopsy (I. S. Roberts et al. 2012). However, postmortem imaging in combination with imaging-guided biopsy seems to hold promise for determining causes of death in patients with comparable accuracy to conventional autopsies, although further studies are necessary (Blokkeret al. 2018; Eriksson et al. 2017).

CONCLUSION

The need for autopsies in improving clinical diagnosis and decision making persists, as recent 20th century studies still show significant discrepancies between clinical diagnoses and findings on autopsy (E. C. Burton, Troxclair, and Iii 1998; Stevanovic et al. 1986; Tai et al. 2001). Indeed, the autopsy and its ability to give definitive answers will continue to be necessary, and may even be expanded to cover other directions. Though the traditional autopsy may have seen its heyday in the 19th and 20th centuries, the autopsy will continue to evolve and be necessary as a tool for medical education, medicolegal purposes, and quality improvement for the near future.

REFERENCES

Aird, W. C. (2011). "Discovery of the Cardiovascular System: From Galen to William Harvey." *Journal of Thrombosis and Haemostasis*, 9 (s1), 118–29. https://doi.org/10.1111/j.1538-7836.2011.04312.x.

Alghamdi, Malak A., Janine, M. Ziermann. & Rui, Diogo. (2017). "An Untold Story: The Important Contributions of Muslim Scholars for the Understanding of Human Anatomy." *The Anatomical Record, 300* (6), 986–1008.

Barr, Justin. (2015). "The Anatomist Andreas Vesalius at 500 Years Old." *Journal of Vascular Surgery, 61* (5), 1370–74.

Bay, Noel Si-Yang. & Boon-Huat, Bay. (2010). "Greek Anatomist Herophilus: The Father of Anatomy." *Anatomy & Cell Biology, 43* (4), 280–83.

Blokker, Britt M., Annick, C. Weustink., Ivo, M. Wagensveld., Jan, H. von der Thüsen., Andrea, Pezzato., Ruben, Dammers., Jan, Bakker., et al. (2018). "Conventional Autopsy versus Minimally Invasive Autopsy with Postmortem MRI, CT, and CT-Guided Biopsy: Comparison of Diagnostic Performance." *Radiology, 289* (3), 658–67.

Breasted, J. H. (1991). *The Edwin Smith Surgical Papyrus, Volume 1: Hieroglyphic Transliteration, Translation, and Commentary|The Oriental Institute of the University of Chicago.*, Vol. *1*, 2 vols. Chicago: The University of Chicago Press.

Burton, Elizabeth C., Dana, A. Troxclair. & William, P. Newman Iii. (1998). "Autopsy Diagnoses of Malignant Neoplasms: How Often Are Clinical Diagnoses Incorrect?" *JAMA, 280* (14), 1245–48.

Burton, Julian L. (2005). "A Bite into the History of the Autopsy." *Forensic Science, Medicine, and Pathology, 1* (4), 277–84.

C. T. E. (1978). "The Earliest Recorded Autopsy in America Performed in 1662 on the 8-Year-Old Elizabeth Kelley." *Pediatrics, 61* (4), 572–572.

Cabot, Richard C. (1912). "Diagnostic Pitfalls Identified During A Study of Three Thousand Autopsies." *Journal of the American Medical Association, LIX* (26), 2295–98.

Campos, Fernando Peixoto Ferraz de. & Luiz, Otávio Savassi Rocha. (2015). "The Pedagogical Value of Autopsy." *Autopsy & Case Reports, 5* (3), 1–6.

Eriksson, Anders., Torfinn, Gustafsson., Malin, Höistad., Monica, Hultcrantz., Stella, Jacobson., Ingegerd, Mejare. & Anders, Persson.

(2017). "Diagnostic Accuracy of Postmortem Imaging vs Autopsy—A Systematic Review." *European Journal of Radiology, 89* (April), 249–69.

Ghosh, Sanjib Kumar. (2015). "Human Cadaveric Dissection: A Historical Account from Ancient Greece to the Modern Era." *Anatomy & Cell Biology, 48* (3), 153–69.

Gulczyński, Jacek., Ewa, Iżycka-Świeszewska. & Marek, Grzybiak. (2009). "Short History of the Autopsy Part I. From Prehistory to the Middle of the 16th Century." *Polish Journal of Pathology, 60* (3), 109–14.

———. (2011). "Short History of the Autopsy: Part II From the Second Half of the 16th Century to Contemporary Times." *Polish Journal of Pathology, 61* (3).

Hadzic, Admir., Neda, Sadeghi., Catherine, Vandepitte., Walter, Vandepitte., Marc, Van de Velde., Alen, Hadzic., Johan, Van Robays., et al. (2014). "500th Birthday of Andreas Vesalius, the Founder of Modern Anatomy: 'Vivitur Ingenio, Caetera Mortis Erunt' ('genius Lives on, All Else Is Mortal')." *Regional Anesthesia and Pain Medicine, 39* (6), 450–55.

Hajar, Rachel. (2012a). "The Air of History: Early Medicine to Galen (Part I)."*Heart Views: The Official Journal of the Gulf Heart Association, 13* (3), 120–28.

———. (2012b). "The Air of History (Part II) Medicine in the Middle Ages." *Heart Views: The Official Journal of the Gulf Heart Association, 13* (4), 158–62.

———. (2013). "The Air of History Part III: The Golden Age in Arab Islamic Medicine An Introduction." *Heart Views: The Official Journal of the Gulf Heart Association, 14* (1), 43–46.

Hoyert, D. L. (2011). "The Changing Profile of Autopsied Deaths in the United States, 1972–2007." In *2011*. Vol. NCHS data brief, no 67. Hyattsville, MD: National Center for Health Statistics. https://www.cdc.gov/nchs/products/databriefs/db67.htm.

King, L. S. & Meehan, M. C. (1973). "A History of the Autopsy. A Review." *The American Journal of Pathology, 73* (2), 514–44.

Menon, I. A. & Haberman, H. F. (1969). "Dermatological Writings of Ancient India." *Medical History, 13* (4), 387–92.

Middendorp, Joost J. van., Gonzalo, M. Sanchez. & Alwyn, L. Burridge. (2010). "The Edwin Smith Papyrus: A Clinical Reappraisal of the Oldest Known Document on Spinal Injuries." *European Spine Journal, 19* (11), 1815–23.

Okuda, Takahisa., Seiji, Shiotani., Namiko, Sakamoto. & Tomoya, Kobayashi. (2013). "Background and Current Status of Postmortem Imaging in Japan: Short History of 'Autopsy Imaging (Ai).'" *Forensic Science International, Postmortem Imaging, 225* (1), 3–8.

Riggs, Christina. (2010). "Funerary Rituals (Ptolemaic and Roman Periods)." In *UCLA Encyclopedia of Egyptology.*, Vol. *1*, 1. https://escholarship.org/uc/item/1n10x347.

Roberts, Charles Stewart. (1990). "The Case of Richard Cabot." In *Clinical Methods: The History, Physical, and Laboratory Examinations*, edited by H. Kenneth Walker, W. Dallas Hall, and J. Willis Hurst, 3rd ed. Boston: Butterworths.

Roberts, Ian S. D., Rachel, E. Benamore., Emyr, W. Benbow., Stephen, H. Lee., Jonathan, N. Harris., Alan, Jackson., Susan, Mallett., et al. (2012). "Post-Mortem Imaging as an Alternative to Autopsy in the Diagnosis of Adult Deaths: A Validation Study." *Lancet, 379* (9811), 136–42.

Savage-Smith, Emilie. (2013). "Medicine In Medieval Islam." In *The Cambridge History of Science*, 139–67. 2. Cambridge: Cambridge University Press. https://doi.org/10.1017/CHO9780511974007.007.

Shojania, Kaveh G. & Elizabeth, C. Burton. (2008). "The Vanishing Nonforensic Autopsy." *New England Journal of Medicine, 358* (9), 873–75.

Stenn, Frederick. (1971). "Six Hundred Years of Autopsies." *Laboratory Medicine, 2* (1), 21–25.

Stevanovic, Gordana., Gordana, Tucakovic., Rajko, Dotlic. & Vladimir, Kanjuh. (1986). "Correlation of Clinical Diagnoses with Autopsy Findings: A Retrospective Study of 2,145 Consecutive Autopsies." *Human Pathology, 17* (12), 1225–30.

Tai, D. Y., El-Bilbeisi, H., Tewari, S., Mascha, E. J., Wiedemann, H. P. & Arroliga, A. C. (2001). "A Study of Consecutive Autopsies in a Medical ICU : A Comparison of Clinical Cause of Death and Autopsy Diagnosis." *Chest, 119* (2), 530–36.

Tweel, Jan G. van den. & Clive, R. Taylor. (2010). "A Brief History of Pathology." *Virchows Archiv, 457* (1), 3–10.

———. (2013). "The Rise and Fall of the Autopsy."*Virchows Archiv, 462* (4), 371–80.

West, John B. (2014). "Galen and the Beginnings of Western Physiology." *American Journal of Physiology-Lung Cellular and Molecular Physiology, 307* (2), L121–28.

Wu, Yi-Li. (2015). "Between the Living and the Dead: Trauma Medicine and Forensic Medicine in the Mid-Qing." *Frontiers of History in China, 10* (1), 38–73.

Zampieri, Fabio., Mohamed, ElMaghawry., Alberto, Zanatta. & Gaetano, Thiene. (2015). "Andreas Vesalius: Celebrating 500 Years of Dissecting Nature." *Global Cardiology Science & Practice*, (5).

In: A Closer Look at Autopsies
Editor: Fernando Robertson

ISBN: 978-1-53617-178-5
© 2020 Nova Science Publishers, Inc.

Chapter 2

MEDICOLEGAL ASPECTS OF THE AUTOPSY

*Akinwumi Oluwole Komolafe**

Department of Morbid Anatomy and Forensic Medicine,
Obafemi Awolowo University, Ile-Ife, Nigeria

ABSTRACT

The autopsy is a major aspect of the practice of medicine which is
used to audit the effectiveness of clinical practice and assist the law
courts in the adjudication of cases in which deaths occurred in suspicious
circumstances in order to guarantee a safe society, prevent secret
homicide, premature deaths and avoid miscarriage of justice. As it
happens with all human endeavours, the practice of medicine is a rich and
variable blend of science and art and as such it is prone to the influence of
human frailties and idiosyncrasies. Many variables affect the conduct,
interpretation and conclusion of the autopsy. Thus, guidelines need to be
put in place to prevent the pathologist from exploiting the circumstances
to an unwholesome advantage of performing below the expected standard
of care with regards to the autopsy. No human is under any compulsion to
always do the needful except there is the watchtower of the law with
untoward consequences and punitive measures for deviants. Therefore it
is imperative for the pathologist to know that his practice of autopsy
pathology and its derivatives such as clinical and forensic autopsies may

* Correspondening Author's Email: akinkomo1@yahoo.com, akinkomolafe@oauife.edu.ng.

be scrutinised by the law courts to ascertain conformity with the standard of care so that his professional opinion does not affect the living through the miscarriage of justice or give a wrong impression as to the cause of death of a deceased person. Such legal scrutiny may be provoked by the decedent's family who may not be pleased by the standard of care at autopsy such as poor presentation of autopsy findings which reflects poor attention to details on the part of the pathologist or outright incompetence. A failure to diagnosis or wrong diagnosis of the cause of death may have a boomeranging effect on the families especially in familial disorders, failure of insurance claims and grievous public health implications for epidemics of infectious diseases. The law therefore continues to keep watch on the specialist in the discipline of anatomical pathology and enables him to maintain appropriate standards in his practice.. Further measures to avoid squabbles with the law and professional hiccups include the pathologist and his supportive staff being absolutely conversant with the jurisdictional requirements of his practice and adhere strictly to such prescriptions except under extenuating circumstances, and even in such situations, anatomical pathologists should make thorough documentation for posterity.

INTRODUCTION

The autopsy or postmortem examination is the systematic dissection of the human body after death with diligent observation of organ changes, integration of the observed changes and appropriate interpretation so as to ascertain the seat of disease, the progression of disease, the extent of the disease and the cause, mechanism, mode and manner of death (Komolafe A.O., Adefidipe A.A., Akinyemi H.A.M. 2018). The postmortem examination is primarily a derivative of the practice of medicine. Medicine itself is a very broad and growing multispecialty practice that can be defined in its all-encompassing nature as any practice engaging the knowledge or application of medical science in skills, competence, expertise, technology in the diagnoses or therapeutic management but not limited to the afore-mentioned; to resolve, address challenges and problems needing such whether it be individual; dead or alive, relations of the dead and living, a group, agency, law court, people, community, country and such like, experimental, clinical trial and translational medicine inclusive. The postmortem examination must therefore engage the knowledge of medical science to answer the questions which prompted the request of the exercise.

The autopsy remains the gold standard in ascertaining the exact cause of death and mechanisms of death and guiding the law court as per the mode and circumstances that initiated the pathophysiological mechanisms that resulted in death (Komolafe A.O., Adefidipe A.A., Akinyemi H.A.M. 2018).

The postmortem examination is divided into two broad categories: clinical or academic autopsies with consent or authorization by the decedent, decedent's family or healthcare surrogate, and medicolegal, coroner's or forensic autopsies governed by extant laws and jurisdictional statutes or duly authorized by the coroner or medical examiner (Komolafe A.O.; Titiloye N.A. 2016). The reasons for the two categories are quite different and therefore the outcomes and the benefits. The hospital autopsy is much for the benefit of the hospital personnel while the medicolegal autopsy is for the benefit of the law courts. However the hospital autopsy may end up as a medicolegal autopsy in which a physician may be accused of manslaughter due to his acts of omission or commission. Clinical autopsies are conducted to provide confirmation, clarification, and ascertain the correctness of antemortem diagnoses (Hooper J.E. and Geller S.A. 2007; Komolafe A.O., Adefidipe A.A. and Akinyemi H.A.M. 2018; Komolafe A.O., Adefidipe A.A., Akinyemi H.A.M. 2018). The clinical autopsies explain organ changes in the light of antemortem clinical information and known clinicopathological progression of diseases. The end result of the clinical autopsy is an autopsy correspondence from the pathologist to the managing physician, stating the highlights of the pathology of the patient, followed up by the comprehensive autopsy report, the questions raised by the autopsy findings as well as the legal implications of the medical care and postmortem findings. The postmortem report and post-autopsy conferences and deliberations with adequate explanation and counselling, provide reassurance to families of the deceased. It is also an avenue to answer their questions regarding the care given and clarify their doubts and disabuse their minds about negative insinuations regarding the management of their departed loved ones. There is also encouragement that previously thought infectious and genetic diseases are not as overtly contagious as believed. Due interaction with relations after the autopsy sessions go a long way to comfort relations that adequate medical care was given and also alleviate ill-feelings of guilt experienced by relations after the death of a loved one.

Postmortem examination is of great importance to the medical and paramedical community, patients' relations and evaluation of hospital standard operation policies, clinical guidelines as well as companies that make electronic diagnostic and therapeutic equipment so as help them to monitor their activities and calibrate them appropriately. Postmortem investigations allow for the audit of the efficacy of new and evolving management guidelines and protocol during clinical trials, evaluation of new diagnostic tests especially rapid bedside tests(point-of-care tests), surgical techniques particularly to assess the effectiveness of less invasive surgeries, devices such as laparoscopic surgeries and drugs especially those used in conservative management (Pakis et al. 2009). The postmortem examination helps to discover contagious infections, heritable disorders, and environmental pollutants, hazardous substances and toxins and other public health epidemiology priorities for the overall benefit of the larger society. Only a diligently conducted autopsy can justifiably prove occupational diseases and guarantee the payment of appropriate compensation and insurance claims (Pakis et al. 2009). The autopsy also provides an extension of medical knowledge and a means to document the health of society by establishing valid mortality statistics. The data obtained may also be used to extrapolate medical knowledge and as an indication of the health of a community, establish genuine morbidity and mortality statistics for budgeting and also assist in epidemiological studies especially in asymptomatic clinico-pathological disorders. The benefits of the autopsy is therefore unquantifiable for all stakeholders in the autopsy process and the implications of the findings and report of the autopsy on the various care givers involved in the management of the case such as the physicians, other healthcare providers, the relations of the deceased and the public health; could have far-reaching consequences on their terms of employment and practice (McCarthy K.M. 1997; Samanta A. and Samanta

J. 2019; Kim C.J. 2014). Despite the interminable benefits of the autopsy, it has virtually disappeared from the menu of the services of many pathology departments with the consequent ripple effects of deficiency in training, skills and competence for pathology trainees, poor feedback to the clinicians and false completion of death certificates among others (Tette E., and Tettey Y. 2014). Turnbull et al. bemoaned the dearth of autopsies in the United Kingdom as they observed and reported a severe fall in UK autopsy rates to critically and abysmally low levels indicating virtual extinction in some UK National Health Trusts (Turnbull A., Osborn M., and Nicholas N. 2015; Turnbull A., Martin J., and Osborn M. 2015). A fundamental teaching, core training and audit tool should not be allowed to die a natural death in the medical curriculum.

The conduct of the autopsy as circumstances permit must be thorough as the findings usually influence future clinical managements and the exercise of meticulous care and due restraint by physicians (Winters et al. 2012; Kuijpers et al. 2014; Eckart et al. 2011; Tejerina et al. 2012). The autopsy because of the diverse interest involved in its request, execution, postmortem ancillary investigations, documentation, reporting and presentation of findings elicits legal intrigues and may be the initiator and the core evidence in legal controversies arising from patients' care.

Important issues about the autopsy include ascertaining the type of the autopsy, clarifying that the proper documents have been obtained and appropriate authentication of requisite forms. Performing the autopsy with relevant photography, archiving of important evidentiary materials such as specimens, clothing, blood stains, and tissue biopsies with preservation of chain of custody is indispensable; if the findings are to be tenable and admissible in a law court (Fryer et al. 2013; Frost et al. 2012). Failure to take critical samples such as blood, hair, urine for toxicology and DNA analysis or do an essential investigation such as histology, histochemical and immunohistochemical stains on tissue after an autopsy session may compromise the veracity of the autopsy report (Bernardi F.D.C., Saldiva P.H.N., and Mauad T., 2005; Roulson J., Benbow E.W., and Hasleton P.S., 2005; Hansen et al. 2014; Skopp G. 2010). Neglect of the crucial medicolegal aspects such as the decedent's biodata, means of identification could also be explored by parties to invalidate the veracity of the autopsy findings and negate the law court's admissibility of medical evidence generated by the autopsy. A pathologist who wilfully assumes that his report of autopsy findings should be admitted by all parties during examination-in-chief and cross examination would be acting presumptuously and of course preposterously. The pathologist is expected by virtue of his training to be an uncompromisable middle-man between the various stakeholders in an autopsy case, no matter the conflicts of interests that his mode of engagement may convey. The pathologist should know that some of the autopsy findings and attempts at interpretation are likely to generate controversies such as auditing the patient's care by the management team on the accepted standard of care, ascertaining a stage to the disease as at the time of death, relating missed findings as crucial to the right diagnosis which was definitely left untreated by the clinicians therefore allowing complications which resulted in death, establishing the immediate cause of death as completely different from the clinicians' previously known pathologies in the patient thus suggesting their low level of competence, establishing that proper medical history was not obtained from the patient or the patient was managed without right interpretation of the symptoms and signs the patient presented with, establishing that incidental findings though unrelated to the cause of death or progression of disease was sadly missed by clinicians and radiologists, establishing an unnecessary intervention on the part of the management team due to improper interpretation of the clinical events in the patient and also establish the clinicopathological basis for atypical presentations which probably misled the manging team to make wrong judgement and execute inappropriate decisions. Clinicians tend to contest issues whenever the postmortem detected cause of death is at variance with known clinico-pathological condition of the patient. A way to avoid medicolegal challenges is for the pathologist never to compromise standards, he needs to take prior history of the cases with rapt attention, question irregularities in stories presented to him, visit the crime scene when necessary in medicolegal cases and always endeavour to perform autopsies in approved places such as autopsy suites in standard health institutions, certified and accredited for the performance of postmortem examinations.

ASPECTS THAT COULD ELICIT MEDICOLEGAL CONSIDERATIONS

The type or class of the postmortem examination is also crucial to the performance, extent of dissection, interpretation and application of the findings. One of the most important things to do before commencing the postmortem examination is to decipher the reasons for the examination in order to answer the main autopsy question. Answering the most crucial autopsy question will guide in the approach to the postmortem examination, techniques to use for the dissection, decide the indispensable documentations crucial to the case. No two autopsy cases are perfectly the same, they may be related and yet with subtle differences and crucial lessons for all to learn. Every case must be considered strictly on its merit even though universal principles are applicable to all autopsies; specific attention should be paid to every case (Komolafe A.O.; Titiloye N.A. 2016, 2009). A routine hospital autopsy may end up as a high profile medicolegal autopsy. It is important for the pathologist to recognise this early and take all necessary precautions to adhere strictly to the standard of care expected for the performance of the class of autopsy (Hugar B.S., Yp G.C. and Harish S 2010). In any confusing medical scenario, the ultimate investigation that answers all questions and clarifies all doubts is the postmortem examination especially if the anatomical pathologist is given the liberty to perform a full dissection in clinical cases. However, not all autopsies can be addressed by just any pathologist. The forensic autopsy is the exclusive preserve of the forensic pathologist to perform due to its highly specialised nature. The medicolegal autopsy is the derivative of the law with a legal seal and mandate empowering the pathologist to use medical knowledge to critically examine corpses and contribute evidence based on medical science to assist legal authorities to take crucial decisions. The forensic autopsy should strive to fulfil the requirements of the law and answer the crucial and relevant legal questions, failure of which questions the pathologist's competence and makes the exercise unprofitable with regards to the law. It is imperative to state that medical evidence is just a portion of a body of evidence in a case. Such postmortem evidence as given by the pathologist is only admissible in the court of law if the findings are consistent with the overall circumstances of the case, justifiably corroborated by other pieces of evidence. Therefore, the medical evidence of the postmortem examination cannot stand in isolation with correlating with other complementary evidence.

Worrisome aspects for clinicians and medical practitioners in investigative cum support departments including radiologists, and pathologists are the fears that postmortem examination may reveal:

Wrong diagnoses such as misdiagnoses, missed diagnoses which include missing a benign or premalignant condition until it becomes malignant. Iatrogenic causes of death could result from bad physician judgement such as physician errors during thoracocentesis (Adeniran A.A., Adegoke O.A., and Komolafe A.O. 2018). Deaths could have been accelerated due to missed primary site of tumour thus compromising the principles of tumour nomenclature thus giving the tumour a wrong name and therefore instituting a wrong mode of management.

The fact that the autopsy is a potential revealer of secrets and a valid method to audit the care given to a patient in reference to the prevailing and acceptable standard of care in an environment compels physicians to abide by protocols and guidelines. The standard of care is the reference that guides both the physician and the decedent's family (patient) in case of fatalities. Thus it behoves pathologists, clinicians and other healthcare providers to be conversant with the aspect of Tort Law governing clinical negligence and medical malpractice so that they adhere to the extant standard of care that most physicians in that speciality and in the prevailing situation would provide. A breach of rules, standards and guidelines could make the families to insinuate negligence and as such request for autopsy should fatalities occur. The pathologist is also not immune to the consequences of wrong conclusions or misleading autopsy diagnoses. Such professional blunders are made when the guiding principles of the interpretation of postmortem findings are neglected (Komolafe A.O. 2018). Such professional blunders may lead to miscarriage of justice (Cordner 2012; Obafunwa J.O., Ajayi O., and Okoye M.I. 2018; Kanchan T. and Krishan K. 2013; Jeffery et al. 2011; Zubair et al. 2012; Hiss J., Freund M., and Kahana T. 2007; Bejesky R. 2013; Qasim A.P., Awan Z.Z., and Ansari A.J. 2016). Postmortem findings may lead to the review of the acceptable standard of care in terms of definitive factors such as clinical practice guidelines, written standard operational policies and guidance, schemes, professional statutes, systematized treatment protocols, standard regulations, specific codes of conduct, operating technique and procedures (Dan et al. 2011; Tette E., Yawson A.E., and Tettey Y. 2014; Veress B. and Alafuzoff I. 1993; Silas et al. 2010; Daramola A.O., Elesha S.O., and Banjo A.A. 2005). Other important though not often considered issues for physicians to remember are religious leanings of patients and relations, traditional, customary and time-honoured practices peculiar to various specialities (Carpenter B. and Tait G. 2010).

Komolafe emphasized that the subject of anatomical pathology seeks solutions by endeavouring to answer questions generated by contextual cases and events with a view to resolve mysteries and clarify controversies and therefore enumerated the following questions as the logical approach to systematic conduct and analyses of the postmortem so as to avoid wrong conclusion (Komolafe A.O. 2018):

a. What are the structural changes observed during autopsies in individual tissues and organs of the body that is identifiable lesions, even when they are just evolving?

b. What disease or disease conditions ae known to impact these structural changes?

c. Are the structural changes in individual tissues and organs of the body related by their causes and effects and anatomical connections of the organs?

d. Can the structural changes in individual tissues and organs of the body be explained by a single disease process or is this a syndrome?

e. What are the evolutionary events from tissue insult to the expressed lesions that is the pathogenesis?

f. What is the pathophysiology? How does this pathological event create abnormal functioning with resultant afflictions in the patient?

g. What unique structural alterations/lesions occur in tissues that pinpoint the initiating disease process that led to the cascade of events?

h. How may we rule out differential diagnoses of the lesions expressed in the tissues in order to resolve the potential conflict of making wrong diagnoses (conflict resolution of overlapping structural changes that may be seen in many diseases?

i. What are the overall attributes of this unique lesion: the morphology (the study of appearances in this case the structure in all entirety? This includes the site of occurrence (location), shape, colour, size (dimensions), consistency, secondary changes among other findings.

j. The stage of the disease process (the extent of the disease) as at the time of death

k. Functional significance or clinical correlation (clinicopathological correlation)

l. The interplay of factors/circumstances that could possibly modify or modulate the disease process. These include co-morbidities, syndromic associations, synchronous, collision and metachronous tumours.

m. What are complications of the disease condition expressed in the index case?

n. What are complications of treatment and interventions as distinct from the complications of the disease process?

o. What are the incidental findings which can be considered minor?

p. What is the exact cause of death indicating the proximate, intermediate and the immediate causes of death?

Changes seen at autopsy depend on the stage of the disease and the expected clinico-pathological expressions and progressive manifestations of the disease process in organ-systems according to the age of the patient at death. The anatomical pathologist owes clinicians and legal authorities the duty of stating the stage or phase of the disease process as at the time of patient's death as one of the following seven categories:

    a.   Predisposing lesion or premalignant disease stage
    b.   Incubation stage or phase
    c.   Evolution stage or phase
    d.   Early stage or phase
    e.   Intermediate stage or phase
    f.   Late stage or phase
    g.   Complicated terminal stage

Patients' death could occur at any of the stages depending on co-morbidities, physicians' interventions, negligence, medical malpractice issues and should be so clearly stated by the pathologist in his report and clinicopathological correlations.

Komolafe also stressed a morphological approach to resolve the challenges encountered during postmortem examination since the postmortem examination is essentially a study of appearances and organ changes in response to disease conditions and conscientiously relating them to specific disease processes or most probable circumstance in which they occurred, having taking time to rule out all conflicting differentials (Komolafe A.O. 2019).

Possible morphologies include (Komolafe A.O.; Titiloye N.A. 2016; Komolafe A.O. 2019):

    a.   Morphology of the disease process that caused the various structural and dysfunctional or pathophysiological changes that resulted in death that is the primary disease or initiating disorder. The initiating event is applicable for a forensic autopsy.

b. Morphology of the predisposing disease condition predating the primary disease process causing death.

c. Morphology of the complications of the primary disease that precipitated the changes and sequence of events resulting in death.

d. Morphology of the complications of treatment.

e. Morphology of the iatrogenic injuries: physicians and other health workers may inflict potentially fatal injuries on patients during diagnostic and therapeutic interventions.

f. Morphology of the syndromic associations: syndromes tend to present as a constellation of lesions that usually occur together. Recognizing syndromes and defining their genetic basis is important for the pathologist so that he does not treat the problems in isolation.

g. Morphology of incidental findings: Incidental findings are chance findings that do not in any way contribute to the disease progression or death. If they contributed to death in any way, then they are not incidental findings. They are then regarded as part of the primary disease process or its complications.

h. Morphology consistent with old age or age related findings. There may be presence of structural changes especially of degenerative nature that could result in death in old age. A change consistent with old age should therefore not be seen as a pathological lesion.

i. Morphologies that constitute non-specific changes and thus inconsequential or inconclusive to be considered as a cause of death or significant to the pathophysiological events that resulted in death.

j. Morphologies of previously healed lesions or relics of previous disease processes. These have no contributions to the pathophysiological events that resulted in death.

The anatomical pathologist is expected by virtue of his training and experience to properly identify lesions, interpret them appropriately and link the changes so as to distinguish one from another and make a clear distinction between all the above morphologic features and relate them carefully, systematically and scientifically to the circumstances of death. Therefore efforts should be made to correlate anatomo-pathological findings with pathophysiology.

It is not in the interest of the physician or managing team to refuse to request for autopsy or to feign that there is no need for one when necessary. Such action then amounts to a breach of duty which may worsen the gravity of an initial breach of duty. An autopsy helps to ascertain the presence and quantify a legally identifiable injury and properly relate the breach to the injury since the breach may incontrovertibly be the proximate cause of the injury, as a basis for appropriation of compensatory damages. Depending on the legal jurisdictions and relevant regulatory council, further punitive damages may be apportioned to the negligent care provider to duly compensate for emotional and psychological trauma, pain and suffering experienced by the patient and the relations (Samanta A. and Samanta J. 2019).

Instances in which medicolegal challenges may arise include:

- Obtaining informed consent about the autopsy
- Proper authorization and certified documents for forensic autopsies
- Extent of performance, proper body reconstruction and body disfigurement
- Organ retention in medical autopsies and forensic autopsies.

INFORMED CONSENT AND AUTHORIZATION OF THE AUTOPSY

While some developing countries may have to employ common law principles in case of autopsy related infringements, most jurisdictions in the United States engage state statutes that state clearly the issues relevant to the autopsy such as authorisation and disposition of organs and corpses. The clinical or academic autopsies need consent from relations of the deceased but the forensic autopsies do not need consent from relations. Rather, authorisation from legal authorities is necessary before the commencement of the autopsy. It is widely accepted only written agreement attached to explanatory and signed documents are valid consent and authorizations. In *Bambrick v Booth Memorial Medical Center*, the court ruled that the defendant was liable for an unauthorized autopsy due to lack of written authorization and rejected the defendants' demurrer of obtaining oral permission. The court noted that the extant statute required written authorization for the permission to be accepted as valid. Strict adherence to statutory constraints is imperative for the pathologist and hospital to avoid litigations and liability.

The issue of obtaining informed consent before examination or performance of any procedure is given the high level of seriousness it deserves. Any physician who deviates from this right to patient's autonomy or their relative to make informed choice about their corpses risks litigations for assault. Though patients who have not approved of autopsy on their corpses may not be in a position to assent to it after death but the next of kin are in vintage position to consent or authorize autopsies. For minors, the parents or guardians can authorize the autopsies. The next of kin may be the spouse, the biological child who knows the indication for the autopsy, the extent of the autopsy and the expectations of the autopsy after the relations have been duly briefed. It is the role of the clinician who initiated the request to gain the consent of the relations after diligent exercise of explanation of the reason; the procedure and issues about sampling of organs and retention of organs have been elucidated. Relations tend to consent to autopsy to a higher degree when all that the procedure entails have ben explained to them (Lynch M.J. 2002; Tsitsikas et al. 2011). In *Foley v Phelps*, the court ruled that the decisions about the postmortem events on the body of the deceased is the sole primary responsibility of the next of kin and autopsy undertaken by medical personnel amounts to violation of the body for which damages could be awarded and constitutes a criminal offence in its actual assessment. The actions of the defendants contravened the subsisting penal code of the State of New York (Phelps 1896). Consent for autopsy also entails the pathologist complying with the extent of permission without giving any excuses whatsoever, even for the so-called advancement of medical science as this will constitute going against the substantive statutes (Carpenter B. and Tait G. 2010).

There is no need for consent for forensic autopsies. The law mandates medicolegal autopsies by its statutes so as to prevent secret homicides and for public health benefits. In virtually all jurisdictions, it is binding on physicians and the general public to refer deaths from suspicious circumstances to the coroner so that he could review the case and possibly set up an inquisition to find out the cause of death (Jeganathan V.S., Walker S.R., and Lawrence C. 2006).

THE ESSENTIALS OF THE FORENSIC AUTOPSY REPORT

After the medicolegal autopsy, issues of appropriate documentation are critical to the admissibility of the report. Findings need to be critically assessed to avoid any miscarriage of justice. The circumstances of death should be clearly and systematically documented. The onus is on the pathologist to obtain and preserve evidence to prove the cause of death and mechanisms of death in relation to the circumstances of death.

The coroner's autopsy report is a potential legal document which is quite sensitive. It betrays the competence or otherwise of the anatomical pathologist, medical practitioner or practicing forensic pathologist who the law sees as a medical expert in this case and whose judgment and opinions carries significant weight in the law court. He may be summoned to court to give evidence-in-chief. The expectation from the anatomical pathologist, medical practitioner or practicing forensic pathologist is thus very great. He is therefore expected to be truthful, unbiased, unassuming, scientific in his judgment, evidence based judgements with no vain extrapolations and avoid contradicting himself.

The main points of a legally sacrosanct coroner's report include the following:

a. Flawless biodata: Flawless biodata is very essential in law for legal reasons. A mistake in biodata documentation may be used to the negative advantage by the defense counsel. It then raises doubt as to whether the postmortem examination was performed on the right corpse.

b. Opening assertive statement: The anatomical pathologist should make a well-guarded and well-constructed opening statement to establish the cause of death consistent with his final opinion with clarity and beyond doubt. Examples include death was due to injuries sustained in a road traffic accident or death was due to natural disease.

c. Simplicity of the language of presentation: Simplify the medical terms into simple lay man's terms as much as possible. Legal authorities would be more comfortable with English words that they can easily relate with.

d. Commensurate general external examination: A clearly supportive general external examination consistent with the overall forensic story and conclusion should be documented in a logical fashion.

e. Ascertain the classic lesions: Define, describe and appropriately document and use classical anatomical landmarks to reference the injuries causing death.

f. Mechanisms of death: State the mechanisms of the injuries so as to establish step-wisely the pathophysiology of the events resulting in death.

g. Critical review and complementary linking of lesions: Link all the lesions seen together scientifically so as to define the circumstances in which the injuries occurred. This is one of the daunting tasks of the anatomical pathologist. It is a product of training, experience, diligence, paying attention to details and growing mental acumen. This is very important because disease and forensic consultations are diverse and do not read books.

h. Diligent search for contributory pathologies: Search diligently for possible contributory lesions or medical ailments to death such as to document the co-morbidities present and their likely contributions or otherwise to the process of death or perhaps the modification of the primary disease process or accelerated its unique progression and unexpected death.

i. Ruling out conflicting differential diagnoses: Consider other diagnoses which the lesions mimic by listing pertinent negatives which includes any other diagnoses that could conflict with your judgment and steps taken to rule them out.

j. Itemise postmortem session diagnostic tests: List any diagnostic tests conducted at autopsy to confirm your suspicions or rule them out.

k. Total laboratory consultation: Include pertinent autopsy histology, clinical chemistry, microbiological and toxicology reports.

l. Absolute documentation of the procedure: Include visual documentation such as photographs or video recording of the postmortem procedure.

The findings should be clearly related together without contradictions and this culminates in an unambiguous conclusion which is the eventual position of the pathologist as an opinion statement about the cause of death, essentially captured as a concise and precise summary of the pathologist's systematic documentation.

It is imperative on the anatomical pathologist and practicing forensic pathologist to be conversant with issues of medicolegal importance on his case and attend to them in his report and also in Evidence-in-Chief in the court of law.

RETENTION OF ORGANS AFTER CLINICAL AND FORENSIC AUTOPSIES

The retention of organs after the postmortem examination is highly contentious and relatives may explore that professional oversight that consent for autopsies do not automatically translate to consent to keep substantial volumes of the organs, other than for diagnostic purposes. In order to avoid possible litigation, it is better to communicate the autopsy procedure and postmortem disposal of organs with the next of kin and gain informed consent after due explanations and answering all questions raised by the next-of-kin. Thereafter the autopsy consent forms and documents should clearly indicate that tissues may be retained for scientific purposes which include relevant investigations and laboratory procedures for proper diagnoses, research, training, teaching, archival and therapeutic purposes. Procedure for the disposal of organs should be clearly stated on the consent forms

THE CONFIDENTIALITY OF THE AUTOPSY REPORT AND PREVENTING UNAUTHORIZED RELEASE OF THE REPORT AND DISSEMINATION OF THE POSTMORTEM FINDINGS

The report from a medical autopsy is handled strictly as a medical record and a medicolegal document. Pathologists should comply with hospital policy regarding medical record privacy. Hospital policy often specifies who may receive a copy of the autopsy report. Generally, the medical records department, the decedent's physician, and various hospital committees receive copies of the report. Statutes may require state agencies to receive copies as well. It may also be in the statutes that autopsy findings be made known to the Division of Public Health Services in the jurisdiction of the pathologist's practice especially with epidemics or highly communicable infectious diseases. In societies where the law permits, there may be room for disclosure under the Freedom of Information Act in public domain as general documents for the benefit of all. However, proper procedures should be followed for such disclosure in order to avoid sanctions for infringement on patient's confidentiality (Komolafe A.O.; Titiloye N.A. 2009). It is the responsibility of the pathologist to protect the integrity of the postmortem report and keep a copy of the report issued in a portable document format (PDF) version in absolute confidentiality. The pathologist may also have a stored electronic version on digital devices or a web-based electronic version for easy recall should be out of the place of routine practice.

THE PIVOTAL PLACE THE AUTOPSY IN MEDICAL MALPRACTICE AND CLINICAL NEGLIGENCE SUITS AND CLAIMS

The central place of the autopsy in medical practice and clinical negligence litigations cannot be overemphasized (Komolafe A.O., Adefidipe A.A., Akinyemi H.A.M. 2018; Zhang et al. 2016). Negligence is failure of action while medical malpractice is inadequate action compared with the standard of care. Though clinicians fear that autopsy may reveal secrets that could lead to litigations, but the autopsy sets records right and does not necessarily increase the risk of medical malpractice. A properly conducted autopsy will allow the defence team of the clinician to explore grounds to exculpate themselves should litigations arise (Komolafe A.O. 2015). A thorough autopsy and clinicopathological correlations will allow the defense team to prepare their case if a lawsuit is filed. Thus, the autopsy helps to disabuse minds of insinuations, rumours, conjectures and wrong conclusions on the sides of the management team and patient's relations. It also helps to argue cases on probabilities and prevent "frivolous claims" regarding the mode of management, progression of disease and the cause of death; therefore mitigating damages if at all any is awarded (Studdert et al. 2006; Puopolo A.L. and Brennan T.A. 2016).

POST-AUTOPSY PRESERVATION OF CORPSE AND RESEARCH ON AUTOPSY SPECIMENS

The preservation of the corpse after the postmortem examination is the responsibility of the pathologist who performed the autopsy. It is very important for the pathologist to dissect the body using a technique that will enable easy reconstruction and access to the body and the organs should a second opinion be required (Connolly et al. 2017). There should be documentation of any harvested organs. Consent should be taken for the relations before organs are kept either for research, presentation for medicolegal reasons or for further investigations or research purposes. It is important to note that embalmment is difficult after full autopsy. It may then be important to do segmental or regional embalmment to prevent decomposition. The pathologist also needs to be conversant with the challenges and difficulties of assaying for chemical substances and other changes that occur in the embalmed body (Savall et al. 2014; Rae et al. 2016; Grabherr et al. 2012). The pathologist should also consider relevant certificates for individual corpse on merit especially for bodies to be repatriated to other countries: death certificate, postmortem report, authorization to remove remains from country where death has occurred, embalming or cremation certificate, status of infection certificate in consonance with universal best practices (Connolly et al. 2017).

THE ROLE OF THE PATHOLOGIST IN INSTITUTIONAL LIABILITY

The acceptance of a patient by a health institution goes with many responsibilities such as a sense of trust in the hospital to protect the rights of the patients. The institutions also have roles to their staff. As much as the hospitals celebrate and identify with the awards of excellence for breakthroughs achieved of their staff, the institutional authorities also should take responsibilities for the liabilities engendered by the malpractice and clinical negligence committed by all categories of staff (Samuels 2018). Employers cannot shy away from the legal doctrine of vicarious liability (Samanta A. and Samanta J. 2019). Procedures carried out by staff must be thoroughly evaluated by the autopsy to determine the techniques, routes of invasion, competence of the staff performing the procedure, the competence of support and axillary staff and the technical competence. The pathologist is not immune to thorough assessment of his competence (Bove K.E., Iery C., and Autopsy Committee, College of American Pathologists 2002; Dettmeyer R., Preuß J., and Madea B. 2004; Allen 2008). The corporate negligence doctrine effectively takes care of hospital liability due to physician malpractice and negligence issues. This is succinctly reflected in *Adamski v Tacoma General Hospital*. In this case, the court held that the hospital is liable for the negligence caused by its physician whatever their schedule of duty or terms of employment as far as they are the agents of the hospital and the relationship between the institution and staff is apparent (Edulla et al. 2016).

Failure to do the bidding of the deceased as specified while alive or as instructed by the next of kin even in end-of-life issues could be a basis for litigation. In *St Elizabeth Hosp v Garrard*, the court established negligence against the hospital for causing emotional distress for the next-of-kin by their failure to perform autopsy as instructed by the next-of-kin.

Failure to take critical samples such as blood, hair, urine for toxicology and DNA analysis or do an essential investigation such as histology, histochemical and immunohistochemical stains on tissue after an autopsy session may compromise the veracity of the report (Bernardi F.D.C., Saldiva P.H.N., and Mauad T. 2005; Roulson J., Benbow E.W., and Hasleton P.S. 2005).

FORENSIC MEDICINE AND PATHOLOGY PRACTICE AS A FALL OUT OF CRIME, MORAL DECADENCE AND SOCIOCULTURAL AND ECONOMIC INTRIGUES

It is the opinion of author based on experience howbeit anecdotal that the premature and violent deaths that prompted the medical examiner's or coroner's request for the expertise of the anatomic pathologist has their basis in the man's sociocultural, socioeconomic problems, pursuits and relationships. The responsibility of the anatomic pathologist goes beyond mere academic presentations in the court of law but rather use his knowledge, practice and expertise to eradicate or at least reduce some criminal activities. Violent and crime related deaths revolve around lust for power, prosperity and untamed passion. Assassinations and deaths by poisoning have occurred due to lust for political power, privileges, partnerships, better placements and development of territorial cultism and gangsters. Property accumulation and lust for prosperity, unbridled covetousness and inordinate desires for gains have led to genocides and bomb explosions. Crime related to passion for the opposite sex is also preponderant. Men have killed others for the purpose of engaging women solely to themselves. Passion for illicit sex has usually ultimately overwhelmed common sense with fatal consequences. For men with unbridled libido, the presence of the oestrogen potentially makes testosterone unstable.

The anatomical pathologist must be thoroughly knowledgeable about his environment, the peculiarities, the prevalent socioeconomic engagements, the local authorities influence as the crime in a place tends to revolve around these factors. The assault weapons are also intimately linked to the financial prowess and equipment used to perform dally tasks. An anatomical pathologist called to an environment must understand the dynamics that modulate crime in that environment so as to be able to answer and address the crucial legal questions. Otherwise he would give an opinion with total disregard of the mode, circumstances and manner of death. This is particularly important in developing countries or "countries with poor resources management sense or skills (CWPRMS)", where the practice of the pathologist may not be backed with appropriate technology or investigate cases to logical conclusion. Most African countries exemplify countries with poor resources management sense as they are interminably bedevilled by poor fiscal policies, poor training schemes for citizens, poor remuneration for specialists, poor health facilities, poor storage facilities for corpses thus making forensic investigations a herculean task, moribund legal systems with obsolete laws and redundant legal procedures, improperly funded police and other law enforcement agents, state organised and managed assassinations, economically-debilitating intertribal wars, retrogressive nepotism, opportunistic, ill-mentored and unprepared political leadership across board who lack programmes for youths who then remain lazy, indecisive, uneducated, jobless, unambitious, aggressive, morally decadent, engage in cultism, gangsterism and assault foreigners; and chronic indebtedness to world powers among other problems. The latter critically strangulates the economies of those countries such that progress in all areas of human endeavours becomes virtually impossible in those countries.

The severe afflictions of the third world countries cannot be separated from their overall forensic pathology experiences.

a. Every crime is a product of compromised morality.

b. Every society gets worse in its indulged crime if no definitive solutions are engaged actively and consistently.

c. There is no first time criminal in court, rather there are habitual criminals caught and brought to the court for the first time.

d. Science is always usually ahead of crime and eventually catches up with crime globally. It is therefore important for the pathologist to keep exhibits for further scientific evaluation to unravel the mysteries in a case rather than close the case premature.

e. The crime scene in every case should be the priority of the pathologist to interrogate carefully. The scene of crime hold relics of the personalities involved, reasons for the crime, the get-away tactics of the criminals among other issues.

f. Every one present in the vicinity of or mentioned in the circumstances of a crime is a potential suspect or contributor and need to cleverly explored in order to avoid misinterpreting a case.

g. Every man is potentially lawless especially if no one is watching and the crime seems eternally covered.

h. Absolute security of any individual, exhibits, document and property is a farce.

i. No one is immune from being compromised in crime, depending on the interests. Every man is potentially ready, capable and prepared to do anything depending on the pressures be it economic, ambition, overriding desires, core values among others. No one should be trusted absolutely to be the sole custodian of evidence. The chain of custody must be legally fool-proof. Duplication of evidence or multiple secured accesses to evidentiary material needs to be put in the hands of individuals with unified and diverse interests. However the principle of vicarious liability holds for the lead anatomical pathologist.

j.   The perpetrators or facilitators of a crime and/or their agents or informants are always in the precinct of the crime, physically or by technology; giving information on the progress of investigation or monitoring to remove, distort or destroy critical evidence.

k.   The closet person to anyone knows the itinerary and so may be the basis of your problems or challenges. The closet persons are usually the most protective or dangerous.

l.   The prevalent or most commonly available weapon is usually the most frequently crime weapon in an environment.

The above involves that all forensic experts work in unison to interrogate a case thoroughly so as to give the best reports to the law courts. It is therefore very clear that the anatomic pathologist cannot practice forensic medicine and pathology without an uncompromised and close working relationship with other forensic experts, as his own evidence is just a portion of a large body of evidence. The anatomical pathologist who practices in an environment without thorough evaluation of the overriding circumstances and peculiar nature, knowledge of the natives' socioeconomic and sociocultural demographics will be a self-conceited, vainly overconfident and overtly theoretical specialist with aberrant opinions and controversial conclusions.

CONCLUSION

The immense role of the autopsy for enlightening on the issues related to death is incontrovertible. Proper designation of autopsies as clinical or forensic autopsies requires appropriate knowledge and training on the part of pathologists, clinicians, and other healthcare providers as well as the crisis management team and medial defense societies and legal teams of healthcare institutions. Legal implications of patients' management modalities and legal considerations of the autopsy findings should be thoroughly considered and included in autopsy discussions and write-ups. Pathologists should be conversant with issues of consent with next-of-kin, authorization, extent of performance, disfigurement, biopsies of specimens, specific organ retention, failure to recognise lesions, link observed findings and diagnose rightly, and unauthorized release of the postmortem report which may amount to contempt of legal authorities or compromise the effective conduct of investigative boards and panels. Pathologists must be aware of the legal aspects of the postmortem examination in order to avoid liabilities for themselves and their healthcare institutions by strict compliance with hospital administrative regulations in clinical autopsies and jurisdictional statutes in forensic autopsies. The fear of medical negligence and malpractice lawsuits based on autopsy performance or non-performance should also be of paramount importance to pathologist, clinicians, radiologist, other healthcare providers and their institutions. The pathologist is duty-bound to perform autopsies according to the prevailing standard of care so that the comprehensive benefits derivable from the postmortem findings are enjoyed by all stakeholders in patients' care. The special nature of the coroner's autopsy as an initiative of law subscribing eminently to medical assistance among other branches of human endeavour is incontrovertible. The pathologist should therefore perform this privileged role in reverence and deference to the law courts. The anatomical pathologist cannot execute this duty as a private duty or exclusive medical duty but rather as a service on behalf of the overriding and supervising authorities, represented by the law courts in this context. The conduct of forensic autopsies as medicolegal service leads to deductions that give weights to legal verdicts.

REFERENCES

Adamski v Tacoma General Hospital, 579 P.2d 970-974 (1978).

Adeniran, A.A., Adegoke, O.O., and Komolafe, A.O. (2018). "Cardiac Tamponade Complicating Thoracocentesis: A Case for Image-Guided Procedure." *Pan African Medical Journal* 29. https://doi.org/10.11604/pamj.2018.29.37.14335.

Allen, T.C. (2008). "Medicolegal Issues in Pathology." *Archives of Pathology & Laboratory Medicine* 132 (2): 186–91. https://doi.org/10.1043/1543-2165(2008)132(186:MIIP)2.0.CO;2.

Bambrick v Booth Memorial Medical Ctr, 593 NYS 2d 252 (NY App Div 1993).

Bejesky, R. (2013). "The Abu Ghraib Convictions: A Miscarriage of Justice." *SSRN Electronic Journal* 32. https://doi.org/10.2139/ssrn.2257060.

Bernardi, F.D.C., Saldiva, P.H.N., and Mauad, T. (2005). "Histological Examination Has a Major Impact on Macroscopic Necropsy Diagnoses." *Journal of Clinical Pathology* 58: 1261–64. https://doi.org/10.1136/jcp.2005.027953.

Bove, K.E., Iery, C., and Autopsy Committee, College of American Pathologists. 2002. "The Role of the Autopsy in Medical Malpractice Cases, I: A Review of 99 Appeals Court Decisions." *Archives of Pathology & Laboratory Medicine* 126 (9): 1023–31. https://doi.org/10.1043/0003-9985(2002)126<1023:TROTAI>2.0.CO;2.

Carpenter, B., and Tait, G. 2010. "The Autopsy Imperative: Medicine, Law, and the Coronial Investigation." *Journal of Medical Humanities* 31 (3): 205–21. https://doi.org/10.1007/s10912-010-9111-7.

Connolly, R., Prendiville R, Cusack, D, and Flaherty, G. 2017. "Repatriation of Human Remains Following Death in International Travellers." *Journal of Travel Medicine.* https://doi.org/10.1093/jtm/taw082.

Cordner, S. 2012. "Forensic Pathology and Miscarriages of Justice." *Forensic Science, Medicine, and Pathology* 8 (3): 316–19. https://doi.org/10.1007/s12024-012-9338-x.

Dan, E.M., Abudu E.K, Umanah, I.N., and Onwuezobe, I.A. 2011. "An Audit of Medical Autopsy: Experience at the University of Uyo Teaching Hospital (UUTH), Niger Delta Region, Nigeria." *Indian Journal of Medical Sciences* 65 (11): 502–9. https://doi.org/http://dx.doi.org/10.4103/0019-5359.109540.

Daramola, A.O., Elesha, S.O., and Banjo, A.A. 2005. "Medical Audit of Maternal Deaths in the Lagos University Teaching Hospital, Nigeria." *East African Medical Journal* 82 (6): 285–89. https://doi.org/ 10.4314/eamj.v82i6.9298.

Studdert, D.M,, Mello, M.M., Gandhi, T.K., Gawande, A.A., Yoon, C., Kachalia, A., and Puopolo, A.L., and Brennan, T.A. 2006. "Claims, Errors, and Compensation Payments in Medical Malpractice Litigation." *The New England Journal of Medicine* 354 (19): 2024–33. https://doi.org/10.1056/NEJMsa054479.

Dettmeyer, R., Preuß, J. and Madea, B. 2004. "Malpractice — Role of the Forensic Pathologist in Germany." *Forensic Science International* 144 (June): 265–67. https://doi.org/10.1016/j.forsciint.2004.04.063.

Eckart, R.E., Shry, E.A., Burke, A.P., McNear, J.A., Appel, D.A., Castillo-Rojas, L.M., Avedissian, L., Pearse L.A., Potter, R.N., Tremaine, L., Gentlesk, P.J., Huffer, L., Reich, S.S. and Stevenson, W.G. 2011. "Sudden Death in Young Adults: An Autopsy-Based Series of a Population Undergoing Active Surveillance." *Journal of the American College of Cardiology* 58 (12): 1254–61. https://doi.org/ 10.1016/j.jacc.2011.01.049.

Edulla, N.K., Ramesh, K., Alugonda, Y., Kothapalli, J. and Goud, A.K.. 2016. "Measure of Liability in Medical Negligence – A Hospital Based Study." *International Archives of Integrated Medicine* 3 (3): 123–27.

Frost, J., Slørdal L., Vege A., and Nordrum I.S. 2012. "Forensic Autopsies in a Naturalistic Setting in Norway: Autopsy Rates and Toxicological Findings." *Forensic Science International* 223 (1–3): 353–58. https://doi.org/10.1016/j.forsciint.2012.10.023.

Fryer, E.P., Traill, Z.C., Benamore, R.E., and Roberts, I.S.D. 2013. "High Risk Medicolegal Autopsies: Is a Full Postmortem Examination Necessary?" *Journal of Clinical Pathology* 66 (1): 1–7. https://doi.org/ 10.1136/jclinpath-2012-201137.

Grabherr, S., Widmer, C., Iglesias, K., Sporkert, F., Augsburger, M., Mangin P. and Palmiere, C. 2012. "Postmortem Biochemistry Performed on Vitreous Humor after Postmortem CT-Angiography."

Legal Medicine 14 (6): 297–303. https://doi.org/10.1016/j.legalmed.2012.04.010.

Hansen, J., Lesnikova, I, Daa Funder, A.M., and Banner, J. 2014. "DNA and RNA Analysis of Blood and Muscle from Bodies with Variable Postmortem Intervals." *Forensic Science, Medicine, and Pathology* 10 (3): 322–28. https://doi.org/10.1007/s12024-014-9567-2.

Hiss, J., Freund, M., and Kahana, T. 2007. "The Forensic Expert Witness-An Issue of Competency." *Forensic Science International* 168 (2–3): 89–94. https://doi.org/10.1016/j.forsciint.2006.06.004.

Hooper, J.E., and Geller, S.A. 2007. "Relevance of the Autopsy as a Medical Tool: A Large Database of Physician Attitudes." *Archives of Pathology and Laboratory Medicine* 131 (2): 268–74.

Hugar, B.S., Yp, G.C, and Harish, S. 2010. "Pattern of Homicidal Deaths." *Journal of Indian Academy of Forensic Medicine* 32 (3): 194–98.

Jeffery, A., Raj, V., Morgan, B., West, K., and Rutty, G.N. 2011. "The Criminal Justice System's Considerations of so-Called near-Virtual Autopsies: The East Midlands Experience." *Journal of Clinical Pathology* 64 (8): 711–17. https://doi.org/10.1136/jclinpath-2011-200008.

Jeganathan, V.S., Walker, S.R., and Lawrence, C. 2006. "Resuscitating the Autopsy in Australian Hospitals." *ANZ Journal of Surgery* 76 (4): 205–7. https://doi.org/10.1111/j.1445-2197.2006.03703.x.

Kanchan, T., and Krishan. K. 2013. "Forensic Pathology – Principles and Overview." In *Encyclopedia of Forensic Sciences*, 193–96. https://doi.org/10.1016/B978-0-12-382165-2.00183-5.

Kim, C.J. 2014. "The Trial of Conrad Murray: Prosecuting Physicians for Criminally Negligent over-Prescription." *American Criminal Law Review* 51 (2): 517–40.

Komolafe, A.O. and Titiloye, N.A. 2009. "The Role of the Pathologist in Medical Litigations." *Nigerian Journal of Postgraduate Medicine* 2 (1): 18–25.

Komolafe, A.O., Titiloye, N.A. 2016. "Essentials of Autopsy Pathology." *Nigerian Journal of Family Practice* 7 (1): 7–14.

Komolafe, A.O., and Titiloye, N.A. 2015. "Litigations in Medical Practice." *Nigeria Journal of Family Practice* 6 (1): 1–4.

Komolafe, A.O. 2019. "The Morphological Basis and Laws of Autopsy Interpretation: Exploring the Relationship between the Basic Medical Sciences, Anatomical Pathology and Clinical Practice." In *Current Trends in Medicine and Medical Research Vol. 4*, edited by Sheriff D.S., 4th ed., 74–79. West Bengal: Book Publisher International. https://doi.org/10.9734/bpi/ctmmr/v4.

Komolafe, A.O. 2018. "Guiding Principles and Laws in the Interpretation of Postmortem Findings." *International Clinical Pathology Journal* 6 (6): 186–90. https://doi.org/10.15406/icpjl.2018.06.00186.

Komolafe, A.O, Adefidipe, A.A, Akinyemi, H.A.M., Ogunrinde, O.V. 2018. "Medical Errors Detected at the Autopsy: A Prelude to Avoiding Malpractice Litigations." *Journal of Advances in Medicine and Medical Research* 27 (7): 1–8.

Komolafe, A.O, Adefidipe, A.A, Akinyemi, H.A.M.. 2018. "Correlation of Antemortem Diagnoses and Postmortem Diagnoses in a Preliminary Survey - Any Discrepancies?" *Nigeria Journal of Family Practice* 9 (1): 105–8.

Kuijpers, C.C.H.J., Fronczek, J., Van De Goot, F.R.W, Niessen, H.W.M., Van Diest, P.W. and Jiwa, M. 2014. "The Value of Autopsies in the Era of High-Tech Medicine: Discrepant Findings Persist." *Journal of Clinical Pathology* 67 (6): 512–19. https://doi.org/10.1136/jclinpath-2013-202122.

Lynch, M.J. 2002. "The Autopsy: Legal and Ethical Principles." *Pathology* 34 (1): 67–70. https://doi.org/10.1080/00313020120105660.

McCarthy, K.M. 1997. "Doing Time for Clinical Crime: The Prosecution of Incompetent Physicians as an Additional Mechanism to Assure Quality Health Care." *Seton Hall Law Review* 28 (2): 569–619.

Obafunwa, J.O., Ajayi, O., and Okoye, M.I. 2018. "Medical Evidence and Proof of Cause of Death in Nigerian Courts." *Medicine, Science and the Law* 58 (2): 122–34. https://doi.org/10.1177/0025802418754576.

Pakis, I., Yayci, N., Karapirli, M., Gunce, E., and Polat., O. 2009. "Autopsy Profiles of Malpractice Cases." *Journal of Forensic and*

Legal Medicine 16 (1): 7–10. https://doi.org/10.1016/j.jflm.2008.05.012.

Phelps, Foley. 1896. *Foley v. Phelps 1,* 551: 1–4.

Puopolo, A.L., and Brennan, T.A. 2016. *Claims, Errors, and Compensation Payments in Medical Malpractice Litigation*, 2024–33.

Qasim, A.P., Awan, Z.A., and Ansari, A.J.. 2016. *Critical Appraisal of Autopsy Work* 10 (4): 194–202.

Rae, G., Husain M., Mcgoey, R. and Swartz, W. 2016. "Postmortem Aortic Dissection: An Artifact of the Embalming Process." *Journal of Forensic Sciences* 61 (January): 246–49. https://doi.org/10.1111/1556-4029.12938.

Roulson, J., Benbow, E.W. and Hasleton, P.S. 2005. "Discrepancies between Clinical and Autopsy Diagnosis and the Value of Post Mortem Histology; a Meta-Analysis and Review." *Histopa-thology* 47 (6): 551–59.

Samanta, A., and Samanta. J. 2019. "Gross Negligence Manslaughter and Doctors: Ethical Concerns Following the Case of Dr Bawa-Garba." *Journal of Medical Ethics* 45 (1): 10–14. https://doi.org/10.1136/medethics-2018-104938.

Samuels, A. 2018. "The Doctor, Negligence and Causation: A Lawyer's Exposition to Doctors, Scientists and Lawyers." *Medicine, Science and the Law* 58 (3): 194–98. https://doi.org/10.1177/0025802418778168.

Savall, F., Dedouit, F., Piercecchi-Marti, M.D., Leonetti, G., Rougé, D. and Telmon, N. 2014. "Acute Aortic Dissection Diagnosed after Embalming: Macroscopic and Microscopic Findings." *Journal of Forensic Sciences* 59 (5): 1423–26. https://doi.org/10.1111/1556-4029.12485.

Silas, O.A., Adoga, A.A., Manasseh, A.N., Echejoh, G.O., Mandong, B.M., and Olu-Silas, R. 2010. "The Role of Necropsy in Diagnostic Dilemmas as Seen in a Tertiary Hospital in North Central Nigeria." *Journal of Tropical Medicine* 2009: 1–3. https://doi.org/10.1155/2009/718984.

Skopp, G. 2010. "Postmortem Toxicology." *Forensic Science, Medicine, and Pathology* 6 (4): 314–25. https://doi.org/10.1007/s12024-010-9150-4.

St Elizabeth Hosp v Garrard, 730 S.W.2d 649 (Tex 1987).

Tejerina, Eva, Esteban, A., Fernández-Segoviano, P., Rodríguez-Barbero, J.M., Gordo, F., Frutos-Vivar, F., Aramburu, J., Algaba, A., García, O.G.S., and Lorente, J.A. 2012. "Clinical Diagnoses and Autopsy Findings: Discrepancies in Critically Ill Patients." *Critical Care Medicine* 40 (3): 842–46. https://doi.org/10.1097/CCM.0b013e3 18236f64f.

Tette, E., Yawson, A.E., and Tettey, Y. 2014. "Clinical Utility and Impact of Autopsies on Clinical Practice among Doctors in a Large Teaching Hospital in Ghana." *Global Health Action* 7 (1): 1–7. https://doi.org/10.3402/gha.v7.23132.

Tsitsikas, D.A., Brothwell, M., Aleong, J.A.C., and Lister, A.T. 2011. "The Attitudes of Relatives to Autopsy: A Misconception." *Journal of Clinical Pathology* 64 (5): 412–14. https://doi.org/10.1136/jcp. 2010.086645.

Turnbull, A., Martin, J and Osborn M. 2015. "The Death of Autopsy?" *The Lancet* 386 (10009): 2141. https://doi.org/10.1016/s0140-6736 (15)01049-1.

Turnbull, A., Osborn, M., and Nicholas, N. 2015. "Hospital Autopsy: Endangered or Extinct?" *Journal of Clinical Pathology* 68 (8): 601–4. https://doi.org/10.1136/jclinpath-2014-202700.

Veress, B., and Alafuzoff, I., 1993. "Clinical Diagnostic Accuracy Audited by Autopsy in a University Hospital in Two Eras." *Quality Assurance in Health Care : The Official Journal of the International Society for Quality Assurance in Health Care* 5 (4): 281–86.

Winters, B., Custer, J., Galvagno, S.M., Colantuoni, E., Kapoor, S.G., Lee, HW., Goode, V., Robinson, K., Nakhasi A., Pronovost, P., and Newman-Toker, D. 2012. "Diagnostic Errors in the Intensive Care Unit: A Systematic Review of Autopsy Studies." *BMJ Quality & Safety* 21 (11): 894–902. https://doi.org/10.1136/bmjqs-2012-000803.

Zhang, K., Li Y., Fan, F., Liu, X., and Deng, Z.H. 2016. "Court Decisions on Medical Malpractice in China after the New Tort Liability Law." *American Journal of Forensic Medicine and Pathology* 37 (3): 149–51. https://doi.org/10.1097/PAF.0000000000000242.

Zubair, S., Tirmizi, A., Mirza, F.H., and Paryar, H.A. 2012. *Medicolegal Investigation of Violent Asphyxial Deaths - An Autopsy Based Study* 6 (3): 86–90.

In: A Closer Look at Autopsies
Editor: Fernando Robertson

ISBN: 978-1-53617-178-5
© 2020 Nova Science Publishers, Inc.

Chapter 3

FROM THE AUTOPSY TABLE TO THE GENETICS BIOTABLE: THE ROLE OF THE PATHOLOGIST INTO THE MOLECULAR GENETIC ERA

Gabriele Margiotta[1,], Emiliano Iacovissi[1], Giuseppe Calvisi[2], Nicoletta D'Alessandris[3] and Pietro Leocata[1]*

[1]University of L'Aquila, Department of Life, Health and Environmental Sciences, L'Aquila, Abruzzo, Italy
[2]"San Salvatore" Civil Hospital of L'Aquila, Section of Surgical Pathology, L'Aquila, Abruzzo, Italy
[3]University of Rome "La Sapienza," Department of Radiological Sciences, Oncology and Anatomical Pathology, Rome, Lazio, Italy

ABSTRACT

In many countries, clinical autopsy rates (i.e., clinical autopsies other than those required by law) have been declining since the 1950s, as a

* Corresponding Author's Email: gabrielemargiotta@hotmail.com.

reflection of a clear trend to reduce the importance of the autopsies. This can be attributed to different causes: overreliance on modern diagnostic research techniques, conflicting beliefs and practices regarding treatment of the dead, or fear of lawsuits if results contradict antemortem diagnosis. But autopsy's utility is incontrovertible. The many benefits of autopsy for patients, families, public health and society include identification of factors of interest to family members. For example, in cases in which a fatal lesion may have had an inherited genetic cause, it may be worthwhile to use tissues (taken during autopsy) for molecular DNA analysis. The findings could be used to counsel the family of the deceased about the risks of inherited disease and about the possible prophylactic measures available. Usually, this practice is defined "molecular autopsy." The first author who used the term "molecular autopsy" was Ackerman in 2001, when he performed a molecular autopsy on a 17-year-old boy found dead in bed. By the date, many studies were conducted for molecular identification of susceptibility genes and mutations involved in sudden cardiac death. In this chapter, we will discuss practical, legal and ethical aspects of this method. The use of autopsy - expecially of the molecular autopsy - results for medical care, education, research, innovation and health administration provides a good motivation for including autopsy and molecular autopsy as important guarantor of safety of patients and their relatives. The early diagnosis by genetic testing will force lifestyle modifications in individuals (the relatives of the deceased) with genetic risk factors, which alone or in combination with other therapeutic options may delay the onset of the disease. New drugs can also be developed using these genes as targets, which may drive the paradigm shift in modern medicine to personalized medicine.

Keywords: molecular autopsy, autopsy rate, sudden cardiac death

INTRODUCTION

The role of forensic pathology is investigating human death in relevance to social risk management to determine the cause of death - especially in violent and unexpected sudden deaths -, which involve social and medicolegal issues. Forensic pathologists respond to social requests through reliable interpretation of these issues in routine casework. In order to do this, pathologists use the autopsy. The term 'autopsy' means, literally, to 'see for oneself'. It includes a detailed external examination and a dissection of organs from the different body cavities – cranial, thoracic, abdominal and pelvic. In a full conventional, non-coronial hospital autopsy, every body cavity is examined in a systematic way to ensure that nothing is missed [1]. This examination is an important source of medical knowledge. The main functions of autopsies are: determination of the cause and manner of death and the underlying medical conditions, teaching tool for medical students and pathologists in training, feedback to clinicians for quality control, source of epidemiological data and for tissue banking, biomedical research tool, source of data for forensic and legal matters, and of documentation for insurance and workers' compensation claims. Classical morphology remains the "gold standard" procedure to investigate deaths, however, with the advent of new promising technologies, updated forensic pathology (involving the application of medical sciences) provides interesting perspectives. In the last few years, a spectrum of ancillary procedures have been developed and incorporated to detail the pathology. Making full use of the available procedures, systematic investigations will allow comprehensive assessment of pathological findings [2].

THE AUTOPSY DECLINE:
WHAT IS HAPPENING IN THE LAST FEW YEARS

The autopsy has been the foundation of pathology training for generations. The nineteenth century saw the heyday of the autopsy, but the twentieth century has seen its subsequent decline. Since 1971, when The Joint Commission no longer required autopsy utilization for hospital accreditation, the number of hospital autopsies in the United States has declined. In this decline several factors have been implicated. Firstly, in the recent time, clinicians do not want autopsies. The reasons offered by clinician doctors for not requesting autopsies are numerous. They range from an aversion for the procedure to a belief that the modern investigative techniques are so accurate that the autopsy can add nothing to the clinical investigations. The increasing clinical confidence in the ante-mortem diagnosis has resulted in fewer autopsies being requested. But there are many studies which show that the discrepancy rate between the cause of death offered by clinicians, when the patient is still alive, and that revealed by the autopsy is 10–30% [3]. In many instances, insufficient priority has been given to autopsies by the same pathologists. At the 2014 meeting of the Association of Pathology Chairs (APC), some pathologists suggested to remove autopsy from the training curriculum of pathology residents, for two reasons: first of all, fewer examination are performed by resident and attending pathologists, bringing as a result some difficulties in providing the number of autopsies required by the American Board of Pathology (ABP) to sit for the basic qualifying examination in anatomic pathology (currently 50 examination), moreover, removal of them from the residency curriculum would provide several additional time for resident training in newer disciplines in pathology, for example informatics or molecular genetics [4]. These changes in medical undergraduate curricula are resulting in many medical students graduating without ever having seen an autopsy. This means that future doctors will have less knowledge of the role of this fundamental examinationin investigating the cause of death, and that they will not have personal experience of this ascertainment to enable them to give informed answers to the concerns of relatives whose agreement is being requested [1].

CAUSES OF DECLINE OF THE AUTOPSY RATE: FINANCIAL AND ADMINISTRATIVE CONSIDERATIONS THAT DRIVE DECISIONS ON DECREASING OF THE REQUESTS OF AUTOPSY

The term "Autopsy rate" refers to the number of deaths receiving an autopsy per all deaths, expressed per 100 deaths. In the last years, in Western Europe, the USA and other parts of the world, autopsy rates have declined markedly. In the USA, they have dropped from approximately 60% in 1950 to less than 5% over the last decade. From 1972 to 2007, they decreased from 16.9% to 4.3% in deaths caused by disease. In the

European region, from 1990 to 2013, autopsy rates decreased less evidently from 23.4% to 20.4%. With so few examinations performed, many conclusions on cause of death are consequently based on diagnoses and tests performed before death, unconfirmed by autoptic exam [5]. The situation is similar elsewhere. There are several causes for decreasing autopsy rates, such as: religious beliefs, pathologists' fear of malpractice litigation, cost of examination, clinicians' lack of interest in this assessment, legal obligations to obtain a consent (usually from relatives), objections to and insufficient knowledge of autopsies among the general public, relatives viewing the autoptic examination as unnecessary, insufficient reimbursement of pathologists, additional workload to clinicians. Some authors hypothesized that pathologists are more interested to new and sophisticated molecular diagnostic tests conducted on tissue biopsies of living patients rather than to autopsy, which has barely changed over the past century [6]. Despite the worldwide decline in autopsy rates, some institutions have succeeded in maintaining a high rate or fighting a declining rate. Elements contributing to this sustained high autopsy rate were: emphasizing to family members the quality-control benefits of unexpected findings, effective organization and integration of all aspects of this examination, quick communication of autoptic findings to clinicians, use of post-mortem examination data in institutional risk management [1].

Which Alternatives to the Autopsy?

If the autopsy rate declines, what are the possible alternatives to post-mortem dissection? Recently, in response to decreased autopsy rates (due to its low acceptability), various noninvasive, or minimally invasive, methods have been developed. These methods, to be effective, should achieve similar results to conventional necropsy. Needle biopsy, endoscopy and radiology for postmortem investigations may be more accepted by family members. However, these analytical techniques are less precise and more expensive than autopsy and require specialized resources. Furthermore, they may provide only partial information and may miss important information. Noninvasive methods, imaging methods such as MRI, computerized axial tomography (virtual autopsy or virtopsy) and ultrasound have also been proposed. The great advantage of these methods is given by the fact that they are noninvasive. For this reason, they are accepted willingly everywhere. But there are some drawbacks. High cost and dependence on sophisticated equipment and specially trained personnel are serious obstacles, particularly in low- and middle-income countries, to widespread introduction of these methods in practice. In addition to these imaging techniques, it is possible to apply Minimally Invasive Autopsy (MIA). It is an important alternative to conventional autopsy. MIA contemplates, using fine biopsy needles, samples of organs, aimed at obtaining tissue fragments for histological and laboristic evaluation. Advantages of this method are simplicity, rapidity, safety and lack of disfigurement. With this method, also, it is possbile to analyse samples for microorganisms. This assessment, with conventional autopsies, is rarely possible, because of the high contamination risk due to the dissection. In spite of everything, MIA still needs to be validated, compared to complete autopsy, and acceptability, feasibility, appropriateness must be evaluated in different geographical, cultural and religious contexts. Some authors have recently published a study aimed at validating whether MIA could replace conventional autopsy for death by natural causes. The authors concluded that minimally invasive autopsy involving biopsy is an interesting perspective, but more research is needed to establish if it is a practical alternative to conventional autopsy [7].

THE ROLE OF THE AUTOPSY IN THE SUDDEN CARDIAC DEATH

An autopsy may reveal noncardiac forms of death: for example, rupture of an aneurysm, pulmonary embolism, advanced tumor. A common cause of sudden death, expecially in young subjects, is sudden cardiac death (SCD). SCD has been defined by the American Heart Association as "the sudden, abrupt loss of heart function in a person who may or may not have been diagnosed with heart disease whereby the time and mode of death are unexpected, and the death occurs either instantly or shortly after symptoms appear." This type of death occurs in structurally normal heart, when a gross and histological examination fails to detect any plausible organic substrate accounting for cardiac arrest ("mors sine materia" or sudden unexplained death), after excluding diseases of the myocardium, great vessels, coronary arteries, valves, and conduction system and non-natural causes of death by toxicology investigation [8]. Previous studies reported that macroscopic heart features were normal in one third of cardiac SCD, even if, in 79% of them, the following histological study revealed pathological substrates (for example, focal myocarditis or cardiomyopathy and conduction system diseases) [8]. In fact, many SCD cases have structural cardiac abnormalities, for example, congenital coronary artery anomalies, hypertrophic cardiomyopathy (HCM), arrhythmogenic right ventricular cardiomyopathy (ARVC), or myocarditis, which are identifiable at autopsy. Despite all, some studies demonstrated that at least 3% and up to 53% of cases of youthful (age 1–35 years) sudden deaths have no morphologic abnormalities at autopsy. These cases are referred to as autopsy-negative sudden unexplained death (SUD) [9].

Sudden unexpected death, particullary of a child or of a young, is devastating for parents and the scientific community, mostly because death is often the first manifestation of the disease. More than 10,000 individuals under the age of 45 years die suddenly and unexpectedly in the USA each year. It is imperative to achieve an identifiable diagnosis, because the lack of a precise diagnosis leaves family members without an explanation for the cause of death of their relative and potentially at risk themselves, even if they have no manifestations of disease [10]: most inherited heart diseases show autosomal dominant inheritance, placing first-degree relatives at 50% risk of harboring a disease-causing variant. But many authors confirmed that a not negligible proportion of SCD in the young (17%) remained unexplained, despite gross and histologic investigations. If this is the case, the traditional tools of morphologic investigation find a barrier in achieving the final diagnosis. In a normal heart, a ventricular fibrillatio can be due to ion channel gene mutations. These observations pushed to molecular biology techniques at postmortem investigation to reach an identifiable diagnosis, followed by mutation screening in first degree relatives to detect healthy carriers at risk [11]. Molecular biology techniques can discover, in the relatives of the deceased person, potentially lethal and heritable channelopathy disorders such as long QT syndrome (LQTS), catecholaminergic polymorphic ventricular tachycardia (CPVT), and Brugada syndrome (BrS). These disorders lead to electrical disturbances in hearts that are structurally normal, and they have the potentiality of instigating electrical abnormalities. These electrical abnormalities are often benign, but can quickly go out of control in a predisposed individual leading to a sudden death. Luckly, thanks to the advances in genetic screening, in the last 15 years the genetic basis of most inherited cardiac arrhythmia disorders has been discovered [9]. These new discoveries are fundamental since fatal inherited primary arrhythmia syndromes, including the long QT syndrome, are not evident in postmortem investigation because they are associated with a structurally normal heart. Some studies in deceased U.S. collegiate athletes [12] and young military personnel [13], revealed a normal heart in a significant proportion of athletes. Finocchiaro and collaborators investigated the causes and circumstances of SCD in a large cohort of athletes, as determined by post-mortem examination performed by an expert cardiac pathologist at the Cardiac Risk in the Young (CRY) center for cardiac pathology in St. George's University of London. In this study, a structurally normal heart accounted for 42% of the overall cohort. The high prevalence in these cohorts underscores the importance of inherited primary arrhythmia syndromes as a major cause of SCD in athletes [14]. In these settings, autopsy may represent the first opportunity to make the proper diagnosis, and the tissue sampling at postmortem for genetic testing may be of help, particularly to solve the puzzle of "mors sine materia" [8]. Molecular genetic testing (also known as molecular autopsy) has provided clues to the cause of death in many SCD cases, when autopsy was inconclusive. Molecular autopsy and clinical evaluation of surviving relatives demonstrate that, at least one third of SCD, are due to lethal arrhythmia attributed to inherited arrhythmia syndromes (IAS) [15].

Furthermore, in some myocardial diseases the border between physiological and pathological changes is poorly defined: for example, fatty infiltration of the right ventricular free wall (frequently misdiagnosed as arrhythmogenic right ventricular cardiomyopathy), athlete's heart with left ventricular hypertrophy or focal myocardial disarray (often misdiagnosed as hypertrophic cardiomyopathy), and scattered focal inflammatory infiltrates (frequently misdiagnosed as myocarditis) [8]. In these cases, the support of molecular genetic testing can lead to a correct diagnosis with more accuracy.

About this point, some guidelines have recommended postmortem cardiac channel genetic testing, specifically when it seems that cardiac channelopathy may be responsible for the sudden death. Unfortunately, due to the timeconsuming and expensive characters of postmortem genetic testing, actually it is necessary, for the forensic pathologist, to be case-selective in requesting a molecular autopsy. Moreover, tissue samples typically collected for the purposes of histopathological analyses are formalin fixed paraffin embedded tissue (FF-PET), because of its easiness of storage and transportation. But, unfortunately, DNA from FF-PET is often error prone and may be unreliable for comprehensive genetic testing. For genetic testing, instead, the best samples to procure highquality DNA include at least 5–10 ml of autopsy blood collected in EDTA tubes, and 5 g of fresh heart, liver, or spleen tissue. These specimens must be stored at − 80 °C until DNA can be extracted. Some authors suggest that 50–100 μl of whole blood on filter paper can also be utilized to extract DNA, but this tends to provide a very small amount of DNA and a limited amount of genetic analysis can be performed with this type of sample [9].

In conclusion, sudden unexpected death (SUD) is devastating for parents. It is particularly stressful to health personnel when no cause is identified after an in-depth analysis including an autopsy and ancillary examinations (toxicology, microbiology, and other analyses). It is very important that guidelines for the procurement of tissue suitable for DNA extraction and analysis be implemented in the standard of care for the postmortem analysis of SUD.

GENETIC KNOWLEDGE OF SCD RELATED DISEASES

Potentially lethal and inheritable arrhythmia syndromes involve electrical disturbances with the ability to produce fatal arrhythmias in a structurally normal heart. These electrical abnormalities have the aptitude to cause the development of a potentially lethal arrhythmia, leading to the sudden death of an otherwise healthy individual [16]. But a lethal arrhytmia can be due also to structural abnormalities of the cardiac muscle causing a progressive loss of electrical stability of the cardiac tissue. The underlying genetic bases responsible for many inherited cardiac arrhythmia syndromes and primary electrical diseases has been discovered and are below summarized.

Inherited Cardiomyopathies

The term "cardiomyopathies" includes a heterogeneous group of disorders that are characterized by structural abnormalities of the cardiac muscle causing a progressive loss of electrical stability of the cardiac tissue through the generation of anatomical arrhythmogenic substrate.

Dilated Cardiomyopathy (DCM)

The prevalence of dilated cardiomyopathy in the general population is likely to be ≥1 in 250 individuals. The transmission is usually autosomal dominant inheritance with reduced penetrance and variable expressivity, but it is also possible autosomal recessive, x-linked or mitochondrial inheritance. Genetically, DCM is the most heterogeneous cardiomyopathy: mutations can involve genes encoding cytoskeletal, nucleoskeletal, mitochondrial, and calcium-handling proteins. To date, more than 50 single genes are linked to inherited DCM, many of them also linked to other lethal and inheritable arrhythmia syndromes [17].

Hypertrophic Cardiomyopathy (HCM)

The prevalence of Hypertrophic cardiomyopathy (HCM) in the general population is one in every 500 people. The transmission is usually the autosomal dominant with variable expressivity and age-related penetrance. To date, around 1,400 mutations in 40 genes have been identified as being responsible for HCM, and about 70% of these mutations are in the sarcomere genes encoding cardiac β-myosin heavy chain (MYH7) and cardiac myosin binding protein C (MYBPC3). Rare X-linked inheritance cases sporadic HCM cases due to de novo mutations in the proband has been reported. Due to the genetic and clinical heterogeneity that characterise HCM, very few genotype–phenotype relationships can be established. The great majority of mutations are unique to each family and there is common to have variable expression of the same or similar mutations with respect to age at presentation, severity of hypertrophy, and prognosis [18].

Arrhythmogenic Right Ventricular Cardiomyopathy (ARVC)

The prevalence of Arrhythmogenic right ventricular cardiomyopathy (ARVC) in the general population is estimated to be 1 in 2000–5000. Genetic studies have identified numerous genes for the disorder; most of these encode components of the cardiac desmosome. Also other genes have been implicated. The majority of mutations involve PKP2 and DSG2, followed by DSP and DCS2. It is common to find low disease penetrance, variable disease expression and severity. Moreover, multiple mutations are found in 6% to 15% of probands, representing in many cases to a more severe phenotype [8].

Primary Electrical Diseases (PED)

Primary electrical diseases (PED) are due to molecular defects in ion channels involved in the generation of the cardiac action potential (AP) and are caused by mutations in genes encoding the cardiac ion channels and their related proteins that cause a 'gain' or a 'loss of function' of one or more ionic currents, resulting in an alteration, during the ventricular AP, of the balance between the depolarizing and repolarizing forces.

Long QT Syndrome (LQTS)

The prevalence of Long QT syndrome (LQTS) in the general population is one in every 2000 people. The transmission is usually inherited in an autosomal dominant manner and classified as Romano-Ward syndrome (RWS), but a rare variant called the Jervell and Lange-Nielsen syndrome (JLNS) is characterized by congenital deafness and autosomal recessive inheritance. Incomplete penetrance is common, and up to 40% of genetic carriers have a normal corrected QT (QTc) interval. Three of the 14 genes associated with LQTS (KCNQ1, KCNH2, SCN5A) account for 70–75% of patients with a definite diagnosis [19].

Brugada Syndrome (BrS)

The prevalence of Brugada syndrome (BrS) in the general population is one in every 2000 people, but it is much higher in Asian and Southeast Asian countries, especially Thailand, Philippines and Japan, reaching 0.5–1 per 1000. The transmission is usually sporadic but, when familial, the condition is inherited as an autosomal–dominant trait with incomplete penetrance. Currently 14 different genes have been identified accounting for most of all inherited BrS cases, but SCN5A, the gene that encodes for the α subunit of the cardiac sodium channel, account for less than 30% of clinically diagnosed BrS patients. Functionally, the majority translate into a loss of function of the cardiac sodium or calcium current, directly or indirectly, or an increase in one of the outward potassium currents [20].

Catecholaminergic Polymorphic Ventricular Tachycardia (CPVT)

The prevalence of Catecholaminergic polymorphic ventricular tachycardia (CPVT) is estimated to be as high as 1 per 10,000. The condition is highly penetrant. Approximately 55–65% of probands carry a mutation in the ryanodine receptor 2 gene (RYR2) which underlies the autosomal dominant form of CPVT. It is also described an autosomal recessive form. In these cases, mutations in the cardiac calsequestrin gene (CASQ2) are described [21].

Short QT Syndrome (SQTS)

The low number of cases reported after 14 years since its description makes Short QT syndrome (SQTS) one of the rarer cardiac channelopathies. The inheritance is autosomal dominant. Even though it is rare, 6 genes have been identified. Three potassium channel genes (KCNH2,KCNQ1,KCNJ2) have been associated with LQTS and SQTS, but while mutations found in the SQTS patients cause a gain of function, the mutations found in LQTS patients cause a loss of the protein function [22].

Other PED

Other rare PED have been associated with mutations in ion-channel genes. These conditions include premature cardiac conduction disease, sinus node disease, early repolarisation syndrome, idiopathic VF, familial atrial fibrillation, and multifocal ectopic Purkinje-related premature contractions [23].

THE TRADITIONAL "MOLECULAR AUTOPSY"

For genetic testing, the best samples to procure highquality DNA include 5–10 ml of autopsy blood collected in EDTA tubes, and 5 g of fresh heart, liver, or spleen tissue. The traditional molecular autopsy has focused on direct DNA sequencing of the protein coding exons of 4 genes, including the three major LQTS genes (KCNQ1, KCNH2, SCN5A) and the CPVT gene (RYR2). Some studies reported detection rates for a disease-causing (pathogenic) mutation of up to 34% of cases, with huge repercussions in the care sector, witnessing the emerging role of this discipline in defining the cause of death and in assisting the relatives of the deceased [24].

THE "EXOME-WIDE MOLECULAR AUTOPSY"

The clinical variability of channelopathy and cardiomyopathy are related to their genetic heterogeneity. The mechanism of genetic heterogeneity is likely polygenic in nature or the effect of environmental factors and genetic mutations in a synergistic fashion. A comprehensive inspection of genes associated with the electrophysiological and contraction functions could help us to understand the molecular mechanisms of these diseases. Exome sequencing is a powerful, high-throughput genomic analysis technology based on the second-generation sequencing platform that is being applied to define the heritability of complex diseases and health-related traits, and it is the most powerful and cost-effective method for the screening of single nucleotide polymorphisms (SNPs) and mutations in the coding genome region [25].

Recent advances in next generation sequencing technologies have allowed ever expanding panels of genes (up to 200 genes) to be re-sequenced from comparatively small quantities of DNA, with excellent throughput capabilities, and in a cost-efficient manner. This includes sequencing the protein coding exons of all 22,000 genes(the "exome"). Thus, next generation sequencing technologies offer the possibility of an "exome-wide molecular autopsy," and allow genetic testing of all major disease-associated genes. Moreover,the exome data can provide information on a number of gene variants for the evaluation of novel disease associations. However, many factors need to be considered in determining the pathogenicity of the dentified variants: for example, the frequency of the variation in genetic population databases, the type of mutation, the type of aminoacid change, the evidence of co-segregation of the variant within a family [26].

In conclusion, High-throughput next-generation sequencing (NGS) technology offers the possibility to identify potentially pathogenic variants. The list of candidate genes involved in SUD has dramatically expanded in the last years because whole exome sequencing (WES) approaches have provided opportunities to explore new genes and other genomic regions of interest [15]. Since the cost of WES is rapidly decreasing, it will become widespread to use next-generation sequencing technology in the evaluation of the cause of death of SUD cases, allowing the use of pathogenic and likely pathogenic variations for cascade testing of surviving family members [25].

DRUGS AND SUDDEN CARDIAC DEATH

It has been said so far that sudden arrhythmic death syndrome (SADS) is a diagnosis of exclusion, defined as a structurally normal heart with no evident abnormality on macroscopic and histological evaluation and a negative result for toxicology screening. However, it is well known that certain drugs prolong the QT duration and might induce Torsades de Pointes in individuals with LQTS. For example, the drugs alimemazine and tomoxetine are known to prolong the QT duration, although the risk for serious cardiovascular adverse events, including significant increases in QTc and sudden cardiac death, is judged to be low. But some studies reported SUD cases with an identified pathogenic LQT variant in patients who were on medication, with therapeutic levels of medicine in the blood toxicology screening.

In conclusions, great caution is advised when considering certain drugs that prolong the QT duration and might induce Torsades de Pointes in individuals with a family history or other known risk factors for cardiovascular disease [26].

THE USE OF FORMALIN FIXED-PARAFFIN EMBEDDED TISSUES FOR MOLECULAR ANALYSIS

The most of the studies about molecular autopsy suggest the use of blood samples or frozen tissue. However, some authors [27] suggest formalin fixed-paraffin embedded tissue (FFPE) as a suitable biological sample for the performance of a molecular autopsy. The potential value of this type of sample is that it can be implemented retrospectively, so it can be possible to investigate also the relatives. In retrospective investigations, preserved tissue is often the only accessible biological sample. Tissue samples are generally collected during an autopsy for the purposes of histopathological analyses, for this reason they undergo preservation processes - formalin fixation and paraffin embedding - which damage nucleic acids. This poses complications for the molecular analyses that can be performed [28]. It would be ideal for the guidelines to suggest, in every case of SUD, to obtain a blood sample for molecular analyses purpose. However, in cases where the autopsy was already performed and cause of death has been not established, a molecular analysis might be performed retrospectively. In these cases, FFPE tissue obtained for histopathology analyses is often available and it can be identified as a biological sample for molecular analysis.

In the near future, with the decreased cost of high throughput sequencing, archived material will represent a valuable resource for translational research. FFPE tissue samples are a potentially valuable resource for retrospective molecular analyses. Actually, the chemical and physical processes during fixation are damaging the quality of DNA obtained, but in a near future various improvements can be made to improve the quality and yield of DNA obtained [28].

LEGAL AND ETHICAL ASPECTS OF MOLECULAR AUTOPSY

Recent advances in the fields of molecular pathology have resulted in the capacity to test for many genetic mutations, fueling the legal issues surrounding forensic autopsy both the prospective analyses of routine cases and the retrospective analyses for research purposes. First of all, in Italy the postmortem examination can be carried out without the consent of the deceased or a proxy. The magistrate can mandate genetic testing on autopsy samples in order to determine the cause of death, but this is not imperative and the decision is frequently referred to the doctor acting as a technical consultant. Conversely, retrospective analyses assimilated to a research activity necessitate consent of the individual prior to death or proxy consent after death, as well as approval by the local ethics committee.

Moreover, genetic testing may cause ethical complications. For instance, the balance between individual privacy versus informing the family members that in a significant percentage of sudden deaths (especially in children and young adults) treatable genetic disorders can be identified. Although medical doctors are not legally bound to inform their patients of the genetic risks of disease, from an ethical standpoint they should inform family members. The doctors must respect the family's wish to know or not to know their genetic predisposition, as expressed during the genetic counseling [29].

Another point to consider is that genetic testing can be performed many years after the death if the samples are properly collected and stored. EDTA blood and a few grams of cardiac or splenic tissues can be stored at −80 °C, limitless. For this reason, appropriate sampling and storage is crucial as well as gathering an appropriate informed consent from who may have the right to it, as well as associating to the sample a reference person for future communications. With the genetic information the clinician has to consider the importance of these data in diagnosis and therapy, risk stratification and management of the SUD family members.

Finally, it is necessary to underline that almost everywhere in the world the law aims to protect individuals who carry morbid genes against discrimination by insurance companies. The latter are not permitted to carry out or require presymptomatic or pre-natal genetic testing before establishing an insurance contract [30].

THE FUTURE OF THE AUTOPSY: WHICH GUIDELINES?

The lack of national or international guidelines for a standardized strategy in SCD cases is the reason why the cause of death remains often undetected. In fact, in the absence of a standard of care, post-mortem examination is still not mandatory in many countries, expert cardiac pathologist is not required in all SCD cases, and the relatives of the victims are not referred for clinical investigations and thereby often undergo incomplete clinical or genetic evaluation. This condition call for development of international guidelines for standardization and centralization of the care for SCD victims and their relatives. The identification of centers of reference on the national territory not only enjoys expertise and knowledge to better deal with the great complexity of genetic cardiac diseases and the psychological issues of the surviving family members, but it possesses also the means to systematically collect the clinical and genetic data in a prospective manner in uniform datasets, which can be aggregated into large national and international registries in homogenous SCD cohorts with large sample sizes. This is essential to ensure accurate research on this topic [31]. In fact, since genetic technology has made DNA sequencing a relatively simple process, and since new genetic alterations underlying inheritable cardiac diseases have been discovered, we are now able to identify novel DNA variants that may cause SCD. The discovery of mutation may also help to improve risk prediction, but it is important to keep in mind that not all the mutations have clinical importance. It is therefore equally important to find ways to distinguish disease-causing mutations from benign variations with no clinical relevance, called "variants of unknown significance" (i.e., VUS). For individuation of these silent variants, it is necessary to standardize the diagnostic approach to SCD to establish a uniform process of genotyping of victims and their relatives. Another measure to be taken is the centralization of the obtained clinical and genetic data in well-structured and homogeneous datasets for future genotype-phenotype correlations [31].

Concluding, standardized guidelines for postmortem investigation of sudden death have not been endorsed in many countries and a blood sample for a molecular autopsy is not always collected. We suggest that a postmortem blood sample and few grams of cardiac or splenic tissues for genetic testing should be kept for all sudden cardiac death. These samples must be placed at -80° until DNA extraction. International scientific societies should fight for mandatory genetic counseling for all cases of sudden cardiac death and for universal guidelines on these topics [27].

THE ROLE PLAYED BY CLINICAL ASSESSMENT OF SURVIVING RELATIVES AND MOLECULAR AUTOPSY IN THE EVALUATION OF SUD: A NEW STANDARD OF CARE? A MULTIDISCIPLINARY COLLABORATION

Cardiac molecular autopsy calls for a close cooperation between many figures: family physician, medical examiner, pathologist, cardiologist, geneticist, and the relatives. Multidisciplinary approach fuels proper genetic counselling of surviving relatives as well as allow for implementing specific preventive or therapeutic strategies, for example, implantation of a implantable cardioverter-defibrillator (ICD) [32]. Fort these reasons, the clinical cardiologic assessment of surviving relatives, combined with a cardiac channel molecular autopsy, should be the standard of care for the postmortem evaluation of SUD [16].

In fact, clinical screening of the family of a case of SUD is most effective if a gene mutation has been found during autopsy, facilitating the clinical evaluation. For this reason interdisciplinary collaboration between different medical disciplines is fundamental for the best management of the affected relatives. Close contact between the involved professional figures is very important. For example, clinical data is often not available for the forensic pathologist, since police investigations focus mainly on criminal circumstances and not in medical assistance [30].

The Next Generation Sequencing technologies will help us to rapidly identify a higher number of genetic variants potentially implicated in arrhythmogenic diseases. This tecnology might be used in routine practice in forensic genetics. Given the massive amount of information generated by NGS, a rigorous filtration strategy is absolutely necessary to facilitate variant classification [33]. However, the following issues limit the usefulness of genetic testing: (a) wide genetic heterogeneity, (b) incomplete penetrance, (c) relatively high frequency of double heterozygotes, and (d) effect of environmental factors [32].

CONCLUSION AND FUTURE DIRECTIONS

The future of autopsy is in the hands of all those who are involved in its continued performance. Pathologists are responsible for obtaining the best results from autopsies and for promoting them.

Autopsy remains essential for pathology training because this practice improves the skills of the operator in any aspect of anatomical pathology practice. For those specialists focused on molecular genetics, remember that post-mortem dissection allows pathologists to procure samples for research in molecular genetics. Without an active necropsy service, this important component of molecular genetic research becomes impossible [34].

Genetic testing must be considered in all equivocal cases. Most of the published genetic guidelines classify genetic testing in case of SADS as useful, and in the case of finding a causative mutation, cascade genetic test is recommended, which means genetic screening in first degree family members [35]. But the family management in these cases is complex and ideally suited for a multidisciplinary specialized approach, including clinical cardiovascular care, genetic evaluation and tests, interpretation of results, conveying the information to the surviving family, and managing the psychosocial wellbeing of the families [24]. This multidisciplinary approach should enable informed genetic counseling for families and should direct the commencement of appropriate preemptive strategies targeted toward averting another tragedy among those left behind [9].

It is of extreme importance that guidelines oriented to the procurement of DNA-friendly sources be added to the standard of care for the postmortem analysis of a SUD. Blood collected in ethylenediaminetetraacetic acid (EDTA) or frozen heart, liver, or spleen provides the greatest source of intact DNA, permitting the successful performance of postmortem cardiac channel genetic testing. 10 ml of EDTA blood or 5 g of fresh tissue should be obtained at autopsy and stored at −80°C, until DNA can be extracted. With rare exceptions, FF-PETs, (i.e., the tissue generally collected during an autopsy for the purposes of histopathological analyses) constitute suboptimal sources for postmortem genetic testing to detect SUD [16].

In conclusion, autopsy remains relevant to medical practice, and therefore, it remains relevant to pathology training. Because autopsy-negative SUD accounts for such a significant number of sudden deaths in the young and considering that cardiac channelopathies contribute to a large portion of these deaths, clinical cardiological assessment of surviving family members and a cardiac channel molecular autopsy should be viewed as the new standard of care for the postmortem evaluation of SUD. The saying "Hic locus est ubi mors gaudet succurrere vitae" remains true.

REFERENCES

[1] Ayoub T, Chow J. The conventional autopsy in modern medicine. *J R Soc Med*. 2008 Apr;101(4):177-81. doi: 10.1258/jrsm. 2008.070479.

[2] Maeda H, Ishikawa T, Michiue T. Forensic molecular pathology: its impacts on routine work, education and training. *Leg Med* (Tokyo). 2014 Mar;16(2):61-9. doi: 10.1016/j.legalmed.2014.01.002. Epub 2014 Jan 17. Review.

[3]   Shojania KG, Burton EC, McDonald KM, et al. Changes in rates of autopsy-detected diagnostic errors over time – A systematic review. *JAMA* 2003;289:2849–56.

[4]   Davis GG, Winters GL, Fyfe BS, Hooper JE, Iezzoni JC, Johnson RL, Markwood PS, Naritoku WY, Nashelsky M, Sampson BA, Steinberg JJ, Stubbs JR, Timmons C, Hoffman RD. Report and Recommendations of the Association of Pathology Chairs' Autopsy Working Group. *Acad Pathol.* 2018 Aug 30;5:2374289518793988. doi: 10.1177/2374289518793988. eCollection 2018 Jan-Dec.

[5]   Hoyert DL. The changing profile of autopsied deaths in the United States, 1972–2007. National Center for Health Statistics. *NCHS Data Brief.* 2011 Aug;(67):1–8.

[6]   Shojania KG, Burton EC. The vanishing nonforensic autopsy. *N Engl J Med.* 2008 Feb 28;358(9):873–5.

[7]   Espinosa-Brito AD, de Mendoza-Amat JH. In Defense of Clinical Autopsy and Its Practice in Cuba. *MEDICC Rev.* 2017 Jan;19(1):37-41.

[8]   Basso C., Bauce B., Corrado D., Thiene G., Pathophysiology of arrhythmogenic cardiomyopathy. *Nat Rev Cardiol,* 2012. 9(4): p. 223-33.

[9]   Boczek NJ, Tester DJ, Ackerman MJ. The molecular autopsy: an indispensable step following sudden cardiac death in the young? *Herzschrittmacherther Elektrophysiol.* 2012 Sep;23(3):167-73. doi: 10.1007/s00399-012-0222-x. Epub 2012 Sep 20.

[10]   Rueda M, Wagner JL, Phillips TC, Topol SE, Muse ED, Lucas JR, Wagner GN, Topol EJ, Torkamani A. Molecular Autopsy for Sudden Death in the Young: Is Data Aggregation the Key? *Front Cardiovasc Med.* 2017 Nov 9;4:72. doi: 10.3389/fcvm.2017.00072. eCollection 2017.

[11]   Thiene G. Sudden cardiac death and cardiovascular pathology: from anatomic theater to double helix. *Am J Cardiol.* 2014 Dec 15;114(12):1930-6. doi: 10.1016/j.amjcard.2014.09.037. Epub 2014 Sep 26. Review.

[12] Harmon KG, Drezner JA, Maleszewski JJ, et al. Pathogeneses of sudden cardiac death in national collegiate athletic association athletes. *Circ Arrhythm Electrophysiol* 2014;7:198–204.

[13] Eckart RE, Shry EA, Burke AP, et al. Sudden death in young adults: an autopsy-based series of a population undergoing active surveillance. *J Am Coll Cardiol* 2011;58:1254–61.

[14] Finocchiaro G, Papadakis M, Robertus JL, Dhutia H, Steriotis AK, Tome M, Mellor G, Merghani A, Malhotra A, Behr E, Sharma S, Sheppard MN. Etiology of Sudden Death in Sports: Insights From a United Kingdom Regional Registry. *J Am Coll Cardiol*. 2016 May 10;67(18):2108-2115. doi: 10.1016/j.jacc.2016.02.062.

[15] Dewar LJ, Alcaide M, Fornika D, D'Amato L, Shafaatalab S, Stevens CM, Balachandra T, Phillips SM, Sanatani S, Morin RD, Tibbits GF. Investigating the Genetic Causes of Sudden Unexpected Death in Children Through Targeted Next-Generation Sequencing Analysis. *Circ Cardiovasc Genet*. 2017 Aug;10(4). pii: e001738. doi: 10.1161/ CIRCGENETICS.116.001738.

[16] Tester DJ, Ackerman MJ. The molecular autopsy: should the evaluation continue after the funeral? *Pediatr Cardiol*. 2012 Mar;33(3):461-70. doi: 10.1007/s00246-012-0160-8. Epub 2012 Feb 4. Review.

[17] Hershberger R. E., Hedges D. J., Morales A., Dilated cardiomyopathy: The complexity of a diverse genetic architecture. *Nat Rev Cardiol*, 2013. 10(9): p. 531-47.

[18] Lopes L. R., Rahman M. S., Elliott P. M., A systematic review and meta-analysis of genotype-phenotype associations in patients with hypertrophic cardiomyopathy caused by sarcomeric protein mutations. *Heart*, 2013. 99(24): p. 1800-11.

[19] Schwartz P. J., Stramba-Badiale M., Crotti L., Pedrazzini M., Besana A., et al., Prevalence of the congenital long-qt syndrome. *Circulation*, 2009. 120(18): p. 1761-7.

[20] Mizusawa Y., Wilde A. A., Brugada syndrome. *Circ Arrhythm Electrophysiol, 2012*. 5(3): p. 606-16.

[21] Hayashi M., Denjoy I., Extramiana F., Maltret A., Buisson N. R., et al., Incidence and risk factors of arrhythmic events in catecholaminergic polymorphic ventricular tachycardia. *Circulation,* 2009. 119(18): p. 2426-34.

[22] Gussak I., Brugada P., Brugada J., Wright R. S., Kopecky S. L., et al., Idiopathic short qt interval: A new clinical syndrome? *Cardiology,* 2000. 94(2): p. 99-102.

[23] Wilde A. A., Behr E. R., Genetic testing for inherited cardiac disease. *Nat Rev Cardiol,* 2013. 10(10): p. 571-83.

[24] Semsarian C, Ingles J. Molecular autopsy in victims of inherited arrhythmias. *J Arrhythm.* 2016 Oct;32(5):359-365. Epub 2015 Nov 19. Review.

[25] Wang C, Duan S, Lv G, Lai X, Chen R, Lin H, Qiu S, Tang J, Kuang W, Xu C. Using whole exome sequencing and bioformatics in the molecular autopsy of a sudden unexplained death syndrome (SUDS) case. *Forensic Sci Int.* 2015 Dec;257:e20-e25. doi: 10.1016/j.forsciint.2015.08.022. Epub 2015 Sep 7.

[26] Stattin EL, Westin IM, Cederquist K, Jonasson J, Jonsson BA, Mörner S, Norberg A, Krantz P, Wisten A. Genetic screening in sudden cardiac death in the young can save future lives. *Int J Legal Med.* 2016 Jan;130(1):59-66. doi: 10.1007/s00414-015-1237-8. Epub 2015 Jul 31.

[27] Bagnall RD, Ingles J, Yeates L, Berkovic SF, Semsarian C. Exome sequencing-based molecular autopsy of formalin-fixed paraffin-embedded tissue after sudden death. *Genet Med.* 2017 Oct;19(10):1127-1133. doi: 10.1038/gim.2017.15. Epub 2017 Mar 23.

[28] Reid KM, Maistry S, Ramesar R, Heathfield LJ. A review of the optimisation of the use of formalin fixed paraffin embedded tissue for molecular analysis in a forensic post-mortem setting. *Forensic Sci Int.* 2017 Nov;280:181-187. doi: 10.1016/j.forsciint.2017.09.020. Epub 2017 Oct 13. Review.

[29] Michaud K, Fellmann F, Abriel H, Beckmann JS, Mangin P, Elger BS. Molecular autopsy in sudden cardiac death and its implication

for families: discussion of the practical, legal and ethical aspects of the multidisciplinary collaboration. *Swiss Med Wkly.* 2009 Dec 12;139(49-50):712-8. doi: smw-12837. Review.

[30] Kauferstein S, Kiehne N, Jenewein T, Biel S, Kopp M, König R, Erkapic D, Rothschild M, Neumann T. Genetic analysis of sudden unexplained death: a multidisciplinary approach. *Forensic Sci Int.* 2013 Jun 10;229(1-3):122-7. doi: 10.1016/j.forsciint.2013.03.050. Epub 2013 Apr 30.

[31] Amin A, Wilde A. The future of sudden cardiac death research. *Progress in Pediatric Cardiology 45* (2017) 49–54.

[32] Hudzik B, Hudzik M, Lekston A, Gasior M. Sudden unexplained cardiac deaths in young adults: a call for multidisciplinary approach. *Acta Cardiol.* 2018 Feb;73(1):7-12. doi: 10.1080/00015385.2017. 1351234. Epub 2017 Jul 26.

[33] Farrugia A, Keyser C, Hollard C, Raul JS, Muller J, Ludes B. Targeted next generation sequencing application in cardiac channelopathies: Analysis of a cohort of autopsy-negative sudden unexplained deaths. *Forensic Sci Int.* 2015 Sep;254:5-11. doi: 10.1016/j.forsciint.2015.06.023. Epub 2015 Jul 3.

[34] Santori M, Blanco-Verea A, Gil R, Cortis J, Becker K, Schneider PM, Carracedo A, Brion M. Broad-based molecular autopsy: a potential tool to investigate the involvement of subtle cardiac conditions in sudden unexpected death in infancy and early childhood. *Arch Dis Child.* 2015 Oct;100(10):952-6. doi: 10.1136/archdischild-2015-308200. Epub 2015 Aug 13.

[35] Brion M, Sobrino B, Martinez M, Blanco-Verea A, Carracedo A. Massive parallel sequencing applied to the molecular autopsy in sudden cardiac death in the young. *Forensic Sci Int Genet.* 2015 Sep;18:160-70. doi: 10.1016/j.fsigen.2015.07.010. Epub 2015 Jul 23. Review.

BIOGRAPHICAL SKETCH

Gabriele Margiotta

Affiliation: University of L'Aquila, Department of Life, Health and Environmental Sciences, L'Aquila, Abruzzo, Italy.

Education: Degree with honors in Medicine at the University of Perugia on Dec. 13, 2005, with a thesis entitled: "Evaluation of allelic alterations in STR in tumors and in formalin-fixed tissues: possible pitfalls in forensic casework." Specialization with honors in Surgical Pathology at the University of L'Aquila on December 16, 2010, with a thesis entitled: "Autopsies at the Institute of Surgical Pathology of L'Aquila in the decade 1999-2008." Specialization with honors in Legal Medicine at the University of Siena on July 11, 2016, with a thesis entitled: ""Validation of a system for forecasting phenotypic traits from traces "

Address: University of L'Aquila, Department of Life, Health and Environmental Sciences, L'Aquila, Abruzzo, Italy. Tel +393883413886.

Research and Professional Experience: Dr. Gabriele Margiotta is interested mostly in Forensic Genetics and Forensic Pathology. He is also interested in paleopathology. He is currently Consultant in Forensic Medicine at the Public Prosecutor's Office of Frosinone, Lazio, Italy.

Publications Last Three Years:
Books:
1. Iacovissi E, Margiotta G., *Principi di Scienza degli Alimenti* [*Principles of Food Science*], Lucisano Editore, 2017, ISBN 978-88-89078-80-8.
2. Iacovissi E., Margiotta G., Anatomia, *Fisiologia e Igiene,* [*Physiology and Hygiene*] Hoepli Editore, 2019, ISBN 978-8820388638

Article:

3. Videtta A, Piccaluga PP, Margiotta G, Santopietro RC, De Falco G. Assessment of clonality of a large cell neuroendocrine carcinoma of the ovary and a well-differentiated neuroendocrine appendix tumour by array-CGH. *Transl Genet Genom* 2017;1:15-26.

In: A Closer Look at Autopsies
Editor: Fernando Robertson

ISBN: 978-1-53617-178-5
© 2020 Nova Science Publishers, Inc.

Chapter 4

ON-SITE TESTING AT FORENSIC AUTOPSY

Hiroshi Kinoshita[1,], Naoko Tanaka[1], Mostofa Jamal[1],
Asuka Ito[1], Mitsuru Kumihashi[1], Tadayoshi Yamashita[1],
Shoji Kimura[1], Yasuhiko Kimura[1], Kunihiko Tsutsui[2],
Shuji Matsubara[3] and Kiyoshi Ameno[1]*

[1]Department of Forensic Medicine, Faculty of Medicine,
Kagawa University, Kagawa, Japan
[2]Health Sciences, Faculty of Medicine,
Kagawa University, Kagawa, Japan
[3]Postgraduate Clinical Education Center,
Kagawa University Hospital, Kagawa, Japan

ABSTRACT

Postmortem biological samples such as blood, urine, bile, tissues, or other materials are collected at forensic autopsy. Various kinds of examinations, including toxicological, microbiological, biochemical, and serological examinations, would be requested from the pathologist. With

---

[*] CorrespondingAuthor: Hiroshi Kinoshita, Department of Forensic Medicine, Faculty of Medicine, Kagawa University, 1750-1, Miki, Kita, Kagawa 761-0793, Japan. E-mail: kinochin@med.kagawa-u.ac.jp.

recent technological developments, some of these examinations can be performed on site, using a single-use device, light portable instruments or examination kits. Since such "on-site" examinations are simple and not time-consuming, the results can be obtained promptly and would be useful for forensic diagnosis.

In the present chapter, on-site examinations at autopsy in forensic practice are discussed.

Keywords: on-site testing, forensic sample, device, examination kit

1. INTRODUCTION

The forensic autopsy has many aims, such as diagnosis of the cause of death, determination of the nature and number of injuries, the presence of poisoning, estimation of the time of death, and personal identification [1]. Forensic pathologist records morphological changes on macroscopic examination, and requires various kinds of ancillary investigations such as biochemical, toxicological, histopathological, and radiological examinations to make a proper diagnosis. Most of the examinations have been traditionally performed on the bench in the laboratory, since the various kinds of examinations have required bench-top equipment and skilled technical staff. Only some of the simple tests, such as urine test strips, have been widely used on-site over the decades.

In recent years, there has been interest in point-of-care testing (POCT) in clinical practice. POCT is defined as diagnostic testing near the patient care environment, and it has been facilitated by the recent development of simple portable devices [2, 3]. Results of POCT are immediately available and provide rapid information to clinicians. Similar to the POCT in clinical practice, various kinds of examinations could be performed at the site of the autopsy. In this paper, the usefulness of on-site examinations in the field of forensic practice is discussed.

2. TYPES OF TESTS AND SAMPLES

The advantage of on-site testing at autopsy is that it provides timely information to the pathologist, which can result in faster and appropriate diagnosis. Single-use devices and portable instruments with an automatic calibration program are widely used in on-site tests. Most tests require no sample preparation and involve ready-to-use reagents. The procedure of on-site testing is usually performed by previously trained technical staff in the autopsy room.

Table 1. On-site test at autopsy

Blood typing
ABO blood typing
Toxicological examination
color test
drug abuse screening panel
CO-oximeter
test tube
test strip
pH in stomach contents
Biochemical analysis
C-reactive protein
HbA1c
other biochemical item
Infectious diseases
immunochromatography for viral infection
(HBs Ag, HCV Ab, HIV Ag/Ab)
other infectious diseases
Immunochromatography
for identification of seminal fluid
identification of human blood
Urine test
test strip

The applicable on-site tests at autopsy are shown in Table 1. Their purposes are personal identification, toxicological screening, pathophysiological examination, and screening for infectious diseases. Specimens such as blood, urine, vitreous humor, cerebrospinal fluid (CSF), gastrointestinal contents, and nasal cavity or pharynx swabs are used. Blood samples at autopsy are routinely obtained from the femoral vein. If peripheral venous blood cannot be obtained, cardiac blood would be used for subsequent investigations. The sampling site of the blood should be recorded in such cases. Urine is obtained by bladder puncture, and care is needed to prevent contamination with blood or other body fluids. The vitreous humor is obtained from the eyeball by needle puncture. CSF is obtained by cisternal puncture or aspirated from the spinal canal following evisceration [4]. The stomach contents are collected in a container at the time the stomach is opened. Liquid from the nasal cavity or pharynx is obtained by a sterile swab supplied with the kit for immunochromatography.

3. TESTS FOR BLOOD TYPING

The ABO blood group system is important in daily forensic practice. Since many people are aware of their ABO blood group and those of close relatives, it is used as one of the items for personal identification. The ABO blood group is defined by the presence or absence of A antigen and B antigen on the surface of red blood cells, and it is distributed differently in various populations [5]. The procedure for ABO blood typing is based on the hemagglutination reaction. Forward (cell) grouping is usually performed on-site at autopsy. Both anti-A antibody (Ab) and anti-B Ab are

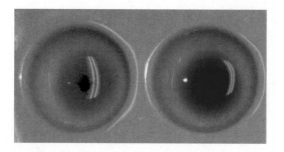

Figure 1. ABO blood typing. Red blood cell aggregates with Anti-A antibody alone (left, blue). This indicates that the blood type is A.

used. A suspension of red blood cells in saline has to be prepared, and one drop each of red blood cell suspension is well mixed with one drop of anti-A Ab and anti-B Ab, respectively, on a plate (plate method), and agglutination is observed. If the red blood cells agglutinate with anti-A Ab alone, the blood type is A (Figure 1). More sensitive blood typing can also be performed in a test tube (tube method).

4. TOXICOLOGICAL EXAMINATION

Rapid identification of drugs and chemicals is important in daily practice [6], as well as in forensic diagnosis.

4.1. Color Test

The color test is rapid and inexpensive and provides information for presumptive identification of drugs and chemicals. It is a simple procedure, and extensive training is not required [7, 8]. Various kinds of color tests have been published [8], and some popular tests are described below.

As a qualitative test for carbon monoxide (CO), a blood sample is mixed with 0.01 M ammonia solution (1:20) [9]. A pinkish tint is observed in the presence of carboxyhemoglobin (CO-Hb). This phenomenon is based on the fact that CO-Hb is relatively tolerant to alkaline conditions. However, since other simple quantitative methods have been established, this color test is rarely required [9].

The urine dithionite test is performed in suspected cases of paraquat and diquat ingestion. Freshly prepared 0.1% sodium dithionite in 1 M sodium hydroxide solution is mixed with 1 ml of urine. A blue or green color indicates the presence of paraquat and diquat [9]. It is a simple and rapid test. To obtain a proper result, a blank (analyte-free) sample using the same matrix as the test sample must be used simultaneously [7]. Subsequent confirmation and quantitation in plasma are required using liquid chromatography [9].

4.2. Screening Panel for Drugs of Abuse

Drug screening tests are widely used in various fields, such as clinical toxicology, forensic toxicology, drug checks at the workplace, and doping inspection, and many drug testing devices have been developed [10-23]. The mainstream on-site drug testing device is an immunoassay. All reagents are included in the kit, and a high skill level or laboratory facilities are not required for the analytical procedure [14]. The Triage® DOA (Biosite Inc., San Diego, CA), one of the commercially available kits, detects eight drug groups such as phencyclidine (PCP), benzodiazepines (BZO), cocaine metabolite (COC), amphetamines (AMP), cannabinoids (THC), opiates (OPI), barbiturates (BAR), and tricyclic antidepressants (TCA) [17, 19]. Another commercially available kit, Instant-View® M-1 (ALFA Scientific Designs, Poway, CA), also detects six drug groups such as methamphetamines (MET), THC, COC, benzodiazepines (BZD), BAR, and TCA [18, 20-23] (Figure 2).

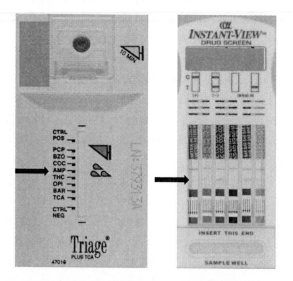

Figure 2. Left: Triage® DOA indicates positive for AMP (amphetamines).
Right: Instant-View® M-1 indicates positive for MET (methamphetamine). (Absence of band shows positive results. And the presence of band shows negative results, even if the band is faint.)

These devices have sufficient sensitivity and specificity for screening, and the result is available within 15 min. However, false-positive results by reaction of the AMP line with phenethylamine in a severely putrefacted sample [13, 17] or tyramine [12], and reaction with ephedrine and its metabolites [24] must be considered. Despite these disadvantages, these devices are quite useful for on-site testing at autopsy, since handling is simple, and multiple drug groups are targeted.

4.3. CO-Oximeter

A CO-oximeter has been used in clinical practice [25-29] and in forensic medicine [30-54]. Original CO-oximeters were large devices only found in the laboratory. However, recently developed portable CO-oximeters can be used for on-site examination. We have been using a portable oximeter, AVOX4000 (AVOX; International Technidyne Corporation, Edison, NJ), which determines various hemoglobin species, such as oxyhemoglobin (O_2-Hb), CO-Hb, methemoglobin (Met-Hb), and total hemoglobin. It automatically indicates the proportion of each species of hemoglobin and oxygen content. This device has many advantages, such as easy handling and portability, requires no sample preparation, and it is suitable for on-site testing (Figure 3).

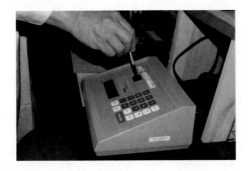

Figure 3. Portable oximeter (AVOX 4000).

Postmortem investigation for CO poisoning or fire-related death is important in forensic practice. CO binds to hemoglobin and forms CO-Hb, which impairs oxygen supply [55]. There is a correlation between clinical symptoms and CO-Hb levels at steady-state concentrations [55]. Severe symptoms such as deep coma or cardiopulmonary failure are observed with a CO-Hb level of around 50%, and CO-Hb levels greater than 50-60% are often fatal [55]. CO-Hb values are important for the diagnosis of CO-poisoning [56]. The quick measurement of CO-Hb using a CO-oximeter provides valuable information for forensic diagnosis.

High levels of Met-Hb have been observed in cases of fire exposure or poisoning by various oxidizing agents such as vehicle exhaust (containing nitric oxide and nitrogen dioxide), nitrate, and chlorate [57-61]. Since Met-Hb impairs O_2 and CO_2 transport, leading to tissue or cellular hypoxia [62], the blood Met-Hb concentration provides useful toxicological information for forensic diagnosis.

Blood in the left cardiac chamber is bright red compared to that in the right cardiac chamber in hypothermic death, and it is one of the characteristic signs of this type of death [37, 38, 52, 54, 63]. The color difference depends on the oxygen content in the blood, and the value of O_2-Hb in cardiac blood obtained by the CO-oximeter is useful for the diagnosis of hypothermic death.

4.4. Test Tube

The detector tube method is widely used for toxicological screening [64-68]. It is also used for quantitation of not only CO, but also cyanide or hydrogen sulfide (H_2S) in blood [64-68]. This apparatus consists of a separator tube, a detector tube, and an aspirating pump connected in series. For CO quantitation, the separator tube (packed silica gel particles coated with ferricyanide) and detector tube (packed sulfite palladium potassium-coated silica gel particles) are used [64-66]. A blood sample (200 µl) is injected into the CO-separator tube, the released CO gas is detected by the CO-detector tube, and it is aspirated by the pump. For cyanide quantitation, different pairs of separator and detector tubes are used. The separator tube is packed silica gel particles coated with sulfuric acid, and the detector tube is packed silica gel particles coated with mercuric chloride and a pH indicator [64, 65, 67]. Hydrogen cyanide (HCN) is released in the separator tube, and hydrochloric acid is formed by the reaction between HCN and mercuric chloride. The H_2S detector tube can also be used for its quantitation in blood [64, 65, 68]. The separator tube for H_2S is packed silica gel particles coated with phosphoric acid, and the detector tube is packed silica gel particles coated with lead acetate [64, 65]. The H_2S gas released in the separator tube is detected by the H_2S-detector tube, followed by aspiration by the pump (Figure 4).

The detector tube method is applied not only for the detection of gaseous substances, but also for the detection of organophosphates, carbamates, salicylates, acetaminophen, or paraquat [65, 69]. Since the detector tube is easy to handle at the scene or at POCT, it is used not only as a screening test, but also for quantitation.

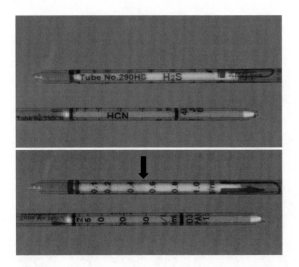

Figure 4. The test tube for hydrogen sulfide (upper part of each picture) and cyanide (lower part of each picture). The blood concentration of hydrogen sulfide is approximately 0.5μg/ml, which is read by the length of discoloration (arrow).

4.5. Test Strip

Test strips are easy to handle and are used to qualitatively test for cyanide and H_2S [69]. The Schöenbein-Pagenstecher method, using guaiac-copper paper, is used as a preliminary test [69]. The guaiac-copper paper turns blue in the presence of cyanide, but must be prepared for use, since it is difficult to store. Another commercially available test paper for cyanide, cyancheck® (ADVANTEC, Tokyo, Japan), is also used for screening [9] (Figure 5).

Lead acetate paper is used as a preliminary qualitative test for H_2S [69, 70]. The sample is mixed with sulfuric acid and heated, and the lead acetate paper turns black in the presence of H_2S. This method is easy, and the result is available quickly [69, 70].

4.6. pH of Stomach Contents

The pH of stomach contents is measured by pH test paper or a handy pH-meter (Figure 5). Since the pH of control postmortem stomach contents ranges from 3.6 to 7.5 [71], a pH value over 7.0 provides useful information for the diagnosis of alkaline solution ingestion, such as cyanide, sodium hydroxide, or potassium hydroxide [72-75].

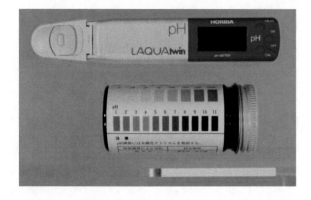

Figure 5. The handy pH-meter (upper) and test strip for cyanide (lower).

5. BIOCHEMICAL EXAMINATION

Biochemical analysis of postmortem blood samples has been applied in daily forensic practice over the last decade [76, 77]. Some of the tests, such as those of potassium and certain enzyme (aspartate aminotransferase (AST), alanine aminotransferase (ALT)) levels in blood, are of little value for postmortem diagnosis [76, 78]. However, some items are stable in the postmortem period and provide reliable results [79].

5.1. C-Reactive Protein (CRP)

C-reactive protein (CRP) is a protein synthesized in the liver in response to inflammatory stimuli, and it is a non-specific marker for immune system activation [80, 81]. Levels of CRP increase during the acute phase response to injury, infection, or other inflammatory stimuli [82, 83]. The procedure for the CRP test is easy, fast, and inexpensive [81], and the CRP level is useful as a forensic marker of inflammation [80]. Its result may aid the pathologist [81].

5.2. HbA1c

Diabetes mellitus (DM) is a disorder of glucose metabolism typically diagnosed based on the casual blood glucose level. However, since the metabolism of glucose continues in the postmortem period, the postmortem blood glucose level is not a reliable marker for the diagnosis of DM in forensic practice.

HbA1c is a glycated hemoglobin formed as a result of non-enzymatic addition of D-glucose [85]. The value of HbA1c depends on mean glucose levels during the 8-12 weeks preceding measurement [84]. It is a reliable marker of DM, and glycated hemoglobin including HbA1c is stable for postmortem sampling [79, 84, 86]. HbA1c is a valuable marker for daily forensic practice [85].

5.3. Other Biochemical Markers

Other biochemical markers such as blood urea nitrogen (BUN), bilirubin, or total cholesterol are also useful for forensic practice [79]. Cardiac troponin T is widely used as a marker for ischemic heart disease in clinical practice [87-90]. Since the postmortem value of cardiac troponin T is affected by various factors, such as postmortem changes and cardiopulmonary resuscitation, cardiac troponin T cannot be used in forensic practice [88, 89].

6. EXAMINATION FOR INFECTIOUS DISEASES

There are many commercially available immunochromatography kits [91-93]. The hepatitis B, hepatitis C, and human immunodeficiency virus antigens or antibodies are easily detected in blood using such kits (Figure 6). From the point of view of biosafety, those results provide useful information in daily practice [94-96].

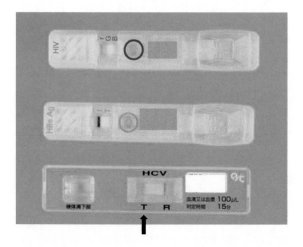

Figure 6. Immunochromatography devices for human immunodeficiency virus, hepatitis B virus and hepatitis C virus antigen or antibody. The antibody for hepatitis C virus is positive (arrow) in the present case.

Respiratory infectious diseases, such as influenza, respiratory syncytial virus (RSV), adenovirus, and human metapneumovirus (hMPV) antigen are detectable by immunochromatography using nasal mucus or pharynx swabs. These positive results provide useful information of the possibility of viral infection prior to the autopsy.

7. OTHER TESTS

7.1. Identification of Seminal Fluid

Prostate-specific antigen (PSA) is a glycoprotein produced by the prostate and secreted into seminal fluid [97, 98]. It is used as an indicator of semen in forensic practice [97-99]. A commercially available immunochromatography PSA kit is used as an on-site testing device in forensic practice (Figure 7). Semenogelin, a protein secreted from seminal vesicles, is used as an alternative method for detection of semen [98]. These kits provide rapid results at the autopsy site.

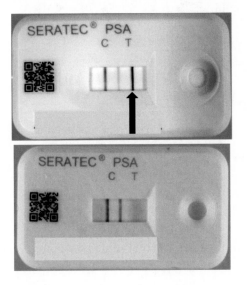

Figure 7. Prostate specific antigen (PSA) test device indicates positive (upper: arrow) and negative reaction (lower).

7.2. Identification of Human Blood

The commercially available fecal occult blood detection kit is applied to differentiate between human and non-human remains. It has high sensitivity for the detection of human hemoglobin [100, 101].

7.3. Urine Test Strip

The urine test strip has been used in daily practice over the last decade [90] (Figure 8). A urine glucose level greater than 25 mg/dL may indicate DM [78]. It is useful for the detection of ketone bodies, which increase in starvation or ketoacidosis. However, if the test strip uses the nitroprusside reaction, it would not react with beta-hydroxybutyrate, which may give a false-negative result in alcoholic ketoacidosis or severe diabetic ketoacidosis [102].

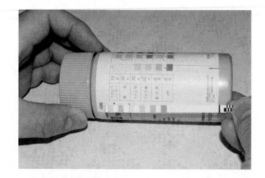

Figure 8. Conventional urine test strip.

CONCLUSION

The data obtained from on-site testing at autopsy are valuable and provide useful information for forensic diagnosis. Further applications of examination kits and development of portable instruments in the fields of forensic practice can be expected.

ACKNOWLEDGMENT

This work was supported by JSPS KAKENHI Grant-in-Aid for Scientific Research (C) Number 18K10127.

REFERENCES

[1] Payne-James, J., Jones, R., Karch, S. B. & Manlove, J. (2011). *Simpson's Forensic Medicine*. London: Hodder Arnold.

[2] Junkar, R., Schlebusch, H. & Luppa, P. B. (2010). Point-of-care testing in hospitals and primary care. *Dtsch Arztebl Int, 107*, 561-567.

[3] Ferreira, C. E. S., Guerra, J. C. C., Slhessarenko, N., Scartezini, M., França, C. N., Colombini, M. P., Berlitz, F., Machado, A. M. O., Campana, G. A., Faulhaber, A. C. L., Galoro, C. A., Dias, C. M., Shcolnik, W., Martino, M. D. V., César, K. R., Sumita, N. M., Mendes, M. E., Faulbhaber, M. H. W., Pinho, J. R. R., Barbosa, I. V., Batista, M. C., Khawali, C., Pariz, V. M. & Andriolo, A. (2018). Point-of-care testing: general aspects. *Clin Lab, 64*, 1-9.

[4] Overfield, J., Dawson, M. & Hamer, D. (1999). *Transfusion Science.* Oxford: Butterworth-Heinemann.

[5] Forrest, A. R. W. (2001). Toxicological and biochemical analysis. In: Burton, JL, Rutty, GN eds. *The hospital autopsy*. pp. 126-133. London: Arnold.

[6] Namera, A. (2009). Simple detection methods for determination of poisons. *Chudoku Kenkyu, 22*, 331-337.

[7] Jeffery, W. & Poole, C. F. (2008). Color tests and thin-layer chromatography. In: Jickells, S, Negrusz A. editors. *Clarke's analytical forensic toxicology*. pp. 335-373. London, Pharmaceutical Press.

[8] Jeffery, W. (2004). Color tests. In: Moffat, AC, Osselton MD, Widdop B. editors. *Clarke's analysis of drug and poisons in pharmaceuticals, body fluids and postmortem materials* (3rd Ed). pp. 279-300. London, Pharmaceutical Press.

[9] Uges, D. R. A. (2004). Hospital toxicology. In: Moffat, AC, Osselton, MD, Widdop, B. editors. *Clarke's analysis of drug and poisons in pharmaceuticals, body fluids and postmortem materials (3rd Ed)*. pp. 3-36. London, Pharmaceutical Press.

[10] Buechler, K. F., Moi, S., Noar, B., McGrath, D., Villela, J., Clancy, M., Shenhav, A., Colleymore, A., Valkirs, G., Lee T., Bruni, J. F., Walsh, M., Hoffman, R., Ahmuty, F., Nowakowski, M., Buechler, J., Mitchell, M., Boyd, D., Stiso, N. & Anderson, R. (1992). Simultaneous detection of seven drugs of abuse by the Triage™ panel for drugs of abuse. *Clin Chem, 38*, 1678-1684.

[11] Wu, A. H. B., Wong, S. S., Johnson, K. G., Callies, J., Shu, D. X., Dunn, W. E. & Wong, S. H. Y. (1993). Evaluation of the triage system for emergency drug-of-abuse testing in urine. *J Anal Toxicol, 17*, 241-245.

[12] Röhrich, J., Schmidt, K. & Bratzke, H. (1994). Application of the novel immunoassay TRIAGE™ to a rapid detection of antemortem drug abuse. *J Anal Toxicol, 18*, 407-414.

[13] Moriya, F. & Hashimoto, Y. (1996). Application of the triageTM panel for drugs of abuse to forensic blood samples. *Nihon Hoigaku Zasshi, 50*, 50-56.

[14] Torre, R. D. L., Domingo-Salvany, A., Badia, R., Gonzàlez, G., McFarlane, D., San, L. & Torrens, M. (1996). Clinical evaluation of the Triage® analytical device for drug-of-abuse testing. *Clin Chem, 42*, 1433-1438.

[15] Peace, M. R., Tarnai, L. D. & Poklis, A. (2000). Performance evaluation of four on-site drug-testing devices for detection of drug of abuse in urine. *J Anal Toxicol, 24*, 589-594.

[16] Mastrovitch, T. A., Bithoney, W. G., DeBari, V. A. & Gold, N. A. (2002). Point-of-care testing for drug of abuse in an urban emergency department. *Ann Clin Lab Sci, 32*, 383-386.

[17] Namera, A., Yashiki, M., Nishida, M. & Kimura, K. (2004). Evaluation of triage for screening of drugs. *Sysmex Journal, 26*, 119-124.

[18] Moody, D. E., Fang, W. B., Andrenyak, D. M., Monti, K. M. & Jones, C. (2006). A comparative evaluation of the Instant-View 5-panel test card with OnTrak TesTcup Pro 5: comparison with gas chromatography-mass spectrometry. *J Anal Toxicol, 30*, 50-56.

[19] Moriya, F. (2008). Advantages and limitation of Triage DOA screening in clinical and forensic drug testing. *Chudoku Kenkyu, 21*, 273-283.

[20] Moriya, F. (2012). Instant-View M-1: a new point-of-care drug testing device. *Chudoku Kenkyu, 25*, 221-226.

[21] Moriya, F., Makino, T., Yoshitome, K., Miura, M. & Miyaishi, S. (2012). Preliminary comparative study on the usefulness of Instant-View™ M-1 and Triage DOA in testing for drugs-of-abuse in forensic urine samples. *Chudoku Kenkyu, 25*, 243-246.

[22] Asano, M., Kuse, A., Morichika, M., Nakagawa, K., Takahashi, M., Kondo, T., Kaszynski, R., Sakurada, M. & Ueno, Y. Evaluation of INSTANT-VIEW™ M-1 for drug abuse screening in judicial autopsies. *Res Pract Forens Med, 55*, 69-77.

[23] Morinaga, M., Okamoto, M., Furukawa, S., Kouguchi, K., Suemori, S. & Tohyama, K. (2016). Basic examination of urinary drug screening kit INSTANT-VIEW M-1. *Japanese Journal of Medical Technology, 65*, 282-289.

[24] Nishiguchi, M., Kinoshita, H., Higasa, K., Taniguchi, T., Ouchi, H., Minami, T., Marukawa, S., Yoshinaga, K., Yamauchi, J., Aoki, S. & Hishida, S. (2001). The false positive reaction of the Triage® panel drug-of-abuse by herbal drugs Ma-huang (*Ephedra sinica (Ephedraceae)*). *Nihon Hoigaku Zasshi, 55*, 331-338.

[25] Zijlstra, W. G., Buursma, A. & Zwart, A. (1988). Performance of an automated six-wavelength photometer (Radiometer OSM3) for routine measurement of hemoglobin derivatives. *Clin Chem, 34*, 149-152.

[26] Mahoney, J. J., Vreman, H. J., Stevenson, D. K. & Van Kessel, A. L. (1993). Measurement of carboxyhemoglobin and total hemoglobin by five specialized spectrophotometers (CO-oximeters) in comparison with reference methods. *Clin Chem, 39*, 1693-1700.

[27] Gong, A. K. (1995). Near-patient measurements of methemoglobin, oxygen saturation, and total hemoglobin: evaluation of a new instrument for adult and neonatal intensive care. *Crit Care Med, 23,* 190-201.

[28] Touger, M., Gallagher, E. J. & Tyrell, J. (1995). Relationship between venous and arterial carboxyhemoglobin levels in patients with suspected carbon monoxide poisoning. *Ann Emerg Med, 25,* 481-483.

[29] Bailey, S. R., Russell, R. N. & Martinez, A. (1997). Evaluation of the avoximeter: precision, long-term stability, and use without heparin. *J Clin Monit, 13,* 191-198.

[30] Okada, M., Okada, T. & Ide, K. (1985). Utilization of a CO-oximeter in the medico-legal field. *Nihon Houigaku Zasshi, 39,* 318-325.

[31] Okada, M., Okada, T., Kawaguchi, N. & Ide, K. (1986). Studies of methemoglobin production in the blood of dead burn victims. *Nihon Houigaku Zasshi, 40,* 124-128.

[32] Ohshima, T., Takayasu, T., Nishigami, J., Lin, Z., Kondo, T. & Nagano, T. (1992). Application of hemoglobin analysis by CO-oximeter to medico-legal practice with special reference to diagnosis of asphyxia. *Nihon Houigaku Zasshi, 46,* 382–388.

[33] Higuchi, T., Noguchi, K. & Maeda, H. (1992). An evaluation of analyzed data of hemoglobin derivatives by CO-oximeter in medico-legal autopsy. *Nihon Houigaku Zasshi, 46,* 416–418.

[34] Maeda, H., Fukita, K., Oritani, S., Nagai, K. & Zhu, B. L. (1996). An evaluation of post-mortem oxymetry in fire victims. *Forensic Sci Int, 81,* 201–209.

[35] Oritani, S., Nagai, K., Zhu, B. L. & Maeda, H. (1996). Estimation of carboxyhemoglobin concentrations in thermo-coagulated blood on a CO-oximeter system: an experimental study. *Forensic Sci Int, 83,* 211–218.

[36] Maeda H., Fukita, K., Oritani, S., Ishida, K. & Zhu, B. L. (1997). Evaluation of post-mortem oxymetry with reference to the causes of death. *Forensic Sci Int, 87,* 201–210.

[37] Shimizu, K., Mizukami, H., Fukushima, T., Sasaki, M. & Shiono, H. (1998). Use of a CO-oximeter for forensic diagnosis of hypothermia. *Nihon Houigaku Zasshi, 52*, 196–201.

[38] Mizukami, H., Shimizu, K., Shiono, H., Uezono, T. & Sasaki, M. (1999). Forensic diagnosis of death from cold. *Leg Med (Tokyo), 1*, 204-9.

[39] Lee, C. W., Tam, J. C. N., Kung, L. K. & Yim, L. K. (2003). Validity of CO-oximetric determination of carboxyhaemoglobin in putrefying blood and body cavity fluid. *Forensic Sci Int, 132*, 153–156.

[40] Brehmer, C. & Iten, P. X. (2003). Rapid determination of carboxyhemoglobin in blood by Oximeter. *Forensic Sci Int, 133*, 179–181.

[41] Watanabe, N., Terazawa, K. & Sakaihara, M. (2003). Blood storage for forensic hemoglobin analysis using CO-oximeter. *Hokkaido Igaku Zasshi, 78*, 289-295.

[42] Watanabe, N. (2003). Medico-legal application of hemoglobin analysis using CO-oximeter. *Hokkaido Igaku Zasshi, 78*, 557-566.

[43] Olson, K. N., Hillyer, M. A., Kloss, J. S., Geiselhart, R. J. & Apple, F S. (2010). Accident or arson: Is Co-oximetry reliable for carboxyhemoglobin measurement postmortem? *Clin Chem, 56*, 515-520.

[44] Tanaka, N., Ameno, K., Jamal, M., Ohkubo, E., Kumihashi, M. & Kinoshita, H. (2010). Application of oximeter AVOX 4000 for the determination of CO-Hb in the forensic practice. *Res Pract Forens Med, 53*, 39-43.

[45] Tanaka, N., Ameno, K., Jamal, M., Kumihashi, M., Kinoshita, H. (2011). Application of oximeter AVOX 4000 in the forensic practice (report 2) –Diagnosis for hypothermia-. *Res Pract Forens Med, 54*, 205-209.

[46] Tanaka, N., Ameno, K., Jamal, M., Kumihashi, M., Miyatake, N. & Kinoshita, H. (2012). Effects of sampling methods and storage on the value of oxyhemoglobin ratio and carboxyhemoglobin ratio. *Res Pract Forens Med, 55*, 51-55.

[47] Kinoshita, H., Tanaka, N., Jamal, M., Kumihashi, M. & Ameno, K. (2012). Evaluation of carboxyhemoglobin (CO-Hb) by oximeter in forensic practice. In: DiLoreto, D, Corcoran, I, editors. *Carbon monoxide source, uses and hazards*. pp. 109-116. New York: Nova Science Publishers, Inc.

[48] Fujihara, J., Kinoshita, H., Tanaka, N., Yasuda, T. & Takeshita, H. (2013). Accuracy and usefulness of the AVOXimeter 4000 as routine analysis of carboxyhemoglobin. *J Forensic Sci, 58,* 1047-1049.

[49] Fujihara, J., Hasegawa, M., Kato, T., Miura, M., Iida, K., Kinoshita, H., Tanaka, N. & Takeshita, H. (2013). A case of drowning lacking typical autopsy findings of carbon monoxide poisoning despite the high CO concentration. *Forensic Toxicol, 31,* 180-182.

[50] Nakagawa, H., Maebashi, K., Fukui, K., Ochiai, E. & Iwadate, K. (2013). Applicability of a new CO oximeter to forensic autopsy cases. *Acta Crim Japon, 79,* 16-21.

[51] Tanaka, N., Ameno, K., Jamal, M., Kumihashi, M., Miyatake, N. & kinoshita, H. (2014). Effects of sample dilution on the value of carboxyhemoglobin ratio. Japanese *Journal of Forensic Pathology, 20,* 39-40.

[52] Kanoto-Nishimaki, Y., Saito, H., Watanabe-Aoyagi, M., Toda, R. & Iwadate, K. (2014). Investigation of oxyhemoglobin and carboxyhemoglobin ratios in right and left cardiac blood for diagnosis of fatal hypothermia and death by fire. *Leg Med (Tokyo), 16,* 321–325.

[53] Tanaka, N., Kinoshita, H., Jamal, M., Takakura, A., Kumihashi, M., Miyatake, N. & Ameno, K. (2015). Squeezed splenic blood sampling as an alternative method for carboxyhemoglobin measurement. *Rom J Leg Med, 23,* 106-108.

[54] Yajima, D., Asari, M., Okuda, K., Maseda, C., Yamada, H., Ichimaru, C., Matsubara, K., Shiono, H., Iwase, H., Makino, Y. & Shimizu, K. (2015). An objective approach using three indexes for determining fatal hypothermia due to cold exposure; statistical analysis of oxyhemoglobin saturation data. *Leg Med (Tokyo), 17,* 451–458.

[55] Elenhorn, M. J. & Barceloux, D. G. (1988). *Medical Toxicology diagnosis and treatment of human poisoning.* New York: Elsevier.

[56] Saukko, P. & Knight, B. (2016). *Knight's forensic pathology.* 4th ed. Boca Raton, FL: CRC Press.

[57] Saito, T., Takeichi, S., Osawa, M., Yukawa, N. & Huang, X. L. (2000). A case of fatal methemoglobinemia of unknown origin but presumably due to ingestion of nitrate. *Int J Legal Med, 113*, 164-167.

[58] Suyama, H., Morikawa, S., Noma-Tanaka, S., Adachi, H., Kawano, Y., Kaneko, K. & Ishihara, S. (2005). Methemglobinemia induced by automobile exhaust fumes. *J Anesth, 19*, 333-335.

[59] Vevelstad, M. & Morild, I. (2009). Lethal methemoglobinemia and automobile exhaust inhalation. *Forensic Sci Int, 187*, e1–e5.

[60] Kinoshita, H., Yoshioka, N., Kuse, A., Nishiguchi, M., Tanaka, N., Jamal, M., Kumihashi, M., Nagasaki, Y., Ueno, Y. & Ameno, K. (2011). A fatal case of severe methemoglobinemia presumably due to chlorate ingestion. *Soud Lek, 56*, 43–44.

[61] Nishiguchi, M., Nushida, H., Okudaira, N. & Nishio, H. (2015). An autopsy case of fatal methemoglobinemia due to ingestion of sodium nitrite. *J Forensic Res, 6*, 262.

[62] Wright, R. O., Lewander, W. J. & Woolf, A. D. (1999). Methemoglobinemia: etiology, pharmacology, and clinical management. *Ann Emerg Med, 34*, 646-656.

[63] Shimizu, K., Shiono, H., Fukushima, T. & Sasaki, M. (1996). Diagnosis of fatal hypothermia –Differences in color between blood from the right and left ventricles and prevalence of Wischnewski's Spot-. *Acta Crim Japon, 62*, 157-160.

[64] Komyo, rikagaku kogyo. (2003). *Gas detector tube system handbook.* 4th ed. Tokyo: Komyo rikagaku kogyo.

[65] Ishizawa, F., Fujita, T., Iseki, K., Hori, T., Saito, T., Usui, K., Hatano, Y., Nozawa, M. & Tominaga, A. (2015). Screening of poisonous substances by detector tube. *Chudoku Kenkyu, 28*, 266-272.

[66] Ishizawa, F. & Misawa, S. (1986). A handy and simple apparatus for the quantitative determination of COHb in blood. *Acta Crim Japon*, *52*, 26-32.

[67] Ishizawa, F. & Misawa, S. (1987). The handy and simple apparatus for the quantitative determination of hydrogen cyanide in blood. *Nihon Houigaku Zasshi*, *41*, 88–92.

[68] Norimine, E., Ishizawa, F., Miyata, K., Ishiwata, T., Yoshida, T. & Honda, K. (2009). Development of detection kit for hydrogen sulfide in blood. *Chudoku Kenkyu*, *22*, 234-235.

[69] Department of Legal Medicine, Hiroshima University. (2001). Simple laboratory procedure of the drug and poisons. Tokyo: Jiho.

[70] Braithwaite, R. A. (2004). Metals and anions. In: Moffat, AC, Osselton, MD, Widdop, B, editors. *Clarke's analysis of drugs and poisons in pharmaceuticals, body fluids and postmortem materials.* pp. 259-278. London: Pharmaceutical Press.

[71] Kamo, K., Tanaka, N., Takakura, A., Jamal, M., Kumihashi, M., Miyatake, N., Tsutsui, K., Kimura, S., Ameno, K. & Kinoshita, H. (2018). The pH value of stomach contents in forensic autopsy cases. *Japanese Journal of Forensic Toxicology*, *24*, 61-63.

[72] Kato, Y., Suzuki, H., Ehara, K., Sato, Y. & Sagisaka, K. (1998). On the autopsy cases in which cyanide were detected in Tokyo Medical Examiner's Office for recent five years. *Res Pract Forens Med*, *41*, 381-386.

[73] Hatake, K., Inoue, T., Morimura, Y., Kudo, R., Fukudome, A., Sageshima, N., Kasuda, S. & Ishitani, A. (2002). An autopsy report of death due to oral ingestion of a rust-preventive agent. *Res Pract Forens Med*, *45*, 51-55.

[74] Satoh, F., Seto, Y., Jin, Z. B., Yukawa, N., Saito, T. & Takeichi, S. (2002). An autopsy case of suicidal ingestion of sodium hydroxide. *Res Pract Forens Med*, *45*, 63-66.

[75] Emoto, Y., Yoshizawa, K., Shikata, N., Tubura, A. & Nagasaki, Y. (2016). Autopsy results of a case of ingestion of sodium hydroxide solution. *J Toxicological Pathol*, *29*, 45-47.

[76] Coe, J. I. (1993). Postmortem chemistry update emphasis on forensic application. *Am J Forensic Med Pathol, 14*, 91-117.

[77] Maeda, H., Ishikawa, T. & Michiue, T. (2011). Forensic biochemistry for functional investigation of death: concept and practical application. *Leg Med (Tokyo), 13*, 55-67.

[78] Kernbach-Wighton, G. & Luna, A. (2014). Postmortem biochemistry as an aid in determining the cause of death. In: Madea B, editor. *Handbook of forensic medicine.* pp. 630-646. West Sussex: John Wiley & Sons, Ltd.

[79] Uemura, K., Shintani-Ishida, K., Saka, K., Nakajima, M., Ikegaya, H., Kikuchi, Y. & Yoshida, K-i. (2008). Biochemical blood markers and sampling sites in forensic autopsy. *J Forensic Leg Med, 15*, 312-317.

[80] Fujita, M. Q., Zhu, B. L., Ishida, K., Quan, L., Oritani, S. & Maeda, H. (2002). Serum C-reactive protein levels in postmortem blood – an analysis with special reference to the cause of death and survival time. *Forensic Sci Int, 130*, 160-166.

[81] Astrup, B. S. & Thomsen, J. L. (2007). The routine use of C-reactive protein in forensic investigations. *Forensic Sci Int, 172*, 49-55.

[82] Young, B., Gleeson, M. & Cripps, A. W. (1991). C-reactive protein: a critical review. *Pathology, 23*, 118-124.

[83] Soejima, M. & Koda, Y. (2014). Evaluation of point-of-care testing of C-reactive protein in forensic autopsy cases. *Forensic Sci Int, 237*, 27-29.

[84] Lepik, D., Tõnisson, M., Kuudeberg, A. & Väli, M. (2018). Glycated haemoglobin (HbA1c) for postmortem diagnosis of diabetes. *Forensic Science Research, 3*, 170-177.

[85] Keltanen, T., Sajantila, A., Valonen, T., Vanhala, T. & Lindroos, K. (2013). Measuring postmortem glycated hemoglobin – a comparison of three methods. *Leg Med (Tokyo), 15*, 72-78.

[86] Kuroda, N. (1990). Determination of glycated hemoglobins of cadaveric blood: a study involving the use of affinity chromatography with m-amino phenyl boronic acid. *Nihon Houigaku Zasshi, 44*, 115–125.

[87] The Joint European Society of Cardiology/American College of Cardiology Committee. (2000). Myocardial infarction redefined – a consensus document of the Joint European Society of Cardiology/ American College of Cardiology comittie for the redefinition of myocardial infarction. *J Am Coll Cardiol, 36*, 959-969.

[88] Davies, S. J., Gaze, D. C. & Collinson, P. O. (2005). Investigation of cardiac troponins in postmortem subjects comparing antemortem and postmortem levels. *Am J Forensic Med Pathol, 26*, 213-215.

[89] Matoba, K., Terazawa, K., Watanabe, S., Yamada, N. & Ueda, M. (2006). Problems in applying rapid assay kit for cardiac troponin T to medico-legal blood samples. *Hokkaido J Med Sci, 81*, 359-363.

[90] Sumita, N. M., Ferreira, C. E. S., Martino, M. D. V., França, C. N., Faulhaber, A. C. L., Scartezini, M, Pinho, J. R. R., Dias, C. M., César, K. R., Pariz, V. M., Guerra, J. C. C., Barbosa, I. V., Faulbhaber, M. H. W., Batista, M. C., Andriolo, A., Mendes, M. E., Machado, A. M. O., Colombini, M. P., Slhessarenko, N., Shcolnik, W., Khawali, C., Campana, G. A., Berlitz, F. & Galoro, C. A. (2018). Clinical applications of point-of-care testing in different conditions. *Clin Lab, 64*, 1105-1112.

[91] Shimetani, N. (2010). Utility and directions of POCT (point of care testing) in diagnosis of infectious disease. *Nihon Rinsho, 68*, supple6, 130-134.

[92] Shimetani, N. (2017). Potential of next-generation POCT in infectious disease rapid test. *Med Mycol J, 58*, J91-J94.

[93] Kozel, T. R. & Burnham-Marusich, A. R. (2017). Point-of-care testing for infectious diseases: past, present and future. *J Clin Microbiol, 55*, 2313-2320.

[94] Otsu, Y., Kibayashi, K., Hamada, K. & Tsunenari, S. (1998). Studies on the positivities of viral infection in forensic autopsy case. *Acta Crim Japon, 64*, 171-175.

[95] Miyaishi, S., Okamura, M., Yamamoto, Y., Yoshitome, K., Ono, T. & Ishizu, H. (1998). Positivities of HBs antigen, anti-HCV antibody and anti-HIV antibody in unnatural death cases. *Japan Medical Journal, 3891*, 42-44.

[96] Tanaka, N., Kinoshita, H., Takakura, A., Jamal, M., Kumihashi, M., Uchiyama, Y., Miyatake, N., Tsutsui, K., Kimura, S. & Ameno, K. (2015). Srudies on the positivity of hepatitis virus and HIV infection in forensic autopsy cases. *Jpn J Forensic Pathology, 21*, 24-26.

[97] Hochmeister, M. N., Budowle, B., Rudin, O., Gehrig, C., Borer, U., Thali, M. & Dirnhofer, R. (1999). Evaluation of prostate-specific antigen (PSA) membrane test assays for the forensic identification of seminal fluid. *J Forensic Sci, 44*, 1057-1060.

[98] Pang, B. C. M. & Cheung, B. K. K. (2007). Identification of human semenogelin in membrane strip test as an alternative method for the detection of semen. *Forensic Sci Int, 169*, 27-31.

[99] Goncalves, A. B. R., de Oliveira, C. F., Carvalho, E. F. & Silva, D. A. (2017). Comparison of the sensitivity and specificity of colorimetric and immunochromatographic presumptive methods for forensic semen detection. *Forensic Sci Int Genet supple Ser6*, e481-e483.

[100] Hochmeister, M. N., Budowle, B., Sparkes, R., Rudin, O., Gehrig, C., Thali, M., Schmidt, L., Cordier, A. & Dirnhofer, R. (1999). Validation studies of an immunochromatographic 1-step test for the forensic identification of human blood. *J Forensic Sci, 44*, 597-602.

[101] Gascho, D., Morf, N. V., Thali, M. J. & Achaerli, S. (2017). The use of immunochromatographic rapid test for tissue remains identification in order to distinguish between human and non-human origin. *Sci Justice, 57*, 165-168.

[102] Nishikawa, M., Shimada, N., Nagayama, I., Fukushima, K., Amano, T., Kawakita, C., Kinomura, M., Asano, K., Kuninaga, N., Fukuoka, T., Ikegami, T. & Fukushima, M. (2014). Pitfalls in the diagnosis of ketoacidosis in the emergency department. *Ann Kurashiki Cent Hospital, 77*, 1-7.

In: A Closer Look at Autopsies
Editor: Fernando Robertson

ISBN: 978-1-53617-178-5
© 2020 Nova Science Publishers, Inc.

Chapter 5

DECLINING AUTOPSY RATES: IS AUTOPSY A DYING PRACTICE?

John L. McAfee and Richard A. Prayson, MD*

Department of Anatomic Pathology, Cleveland Clinic,
Cleveland, OH, US

ABSTRACT

The importance of performing autopsies has been recognized for centuries. Despite this, autopsy rates in the last several decades have dramatically fallen off. This chapter explores the myriad aspects that may be contributing to this downward trend. Many clinicians feel uncomfortable requesting autopsies. Many of these same clinicians have never seen an autopsy performed; it is not a requirement of medical school education anymore. Many clinicians operate under the false assumption that with modern technology, autopsies do not add anything and are obsolete. In fact, the rates of missed diagnoses found at autopsy have not changed dramatically, despite these advances in technology. There is also a fear that findings uncovered at autopsy may be used as medicolegal weapons against the physician caregiver. Pathologists who perform autopsies find it a burden, particularly since there is no financial compensation for performing them. Although hospitals pay lip service to

* Corresponding Author Email: praysor@ccf.org.

autopsies' importance as a quality control measure, they too see autopsies as a money loser.

INTRODUCTION

The percentages of patients who undergo postmortem examination have been falling around the world for several decades. This decline in autopsy rates has been extensively described in the primary literature [1-21]. It has also received regular review and commentary by pathologists and other physicians [22-45]. Many factors may be contributing to this trend; these range from individual decisions, such as whether or not an autopsy is requested or declined, all the way up to institutional and national policies. Autopsies offer numerous benefits to the family of the individual, to physicians who took care of the individual, as well as to the populations who may be affected by certain disease processes. Just as autopsies may provide a patient's family with new information and peace of mind, they may also inform national disease trends and statistics. All of these benefits are missed, when autopsies are not performed in meaningful numbers. A relatively small number of prospective studies have attempted to combat falling autopsy rates and have met some success.

The goal of this chapter is to review the literature relevant to these topics. We will examine the data regarding falling rates and break it down into causes and contributing factors when possible. We will also describe a number of the problems with declining autopsy rates and highlight potential interventions. Through this discussion, we will focus on the hospital or medical autopsy, addressing medical-legal or forensic autopsies only as they relate to specific facets of the published data.

THE DECLINE IN AUTOPSY RATES

A large number of studies from many countries document falling medical autopsy rates on the national level. A United States Centers for Disease Control and Prevention data brief reflected a national decline from

19.3% to 8.5% between 1972 and 2007. The proportion of these autopsies performed for medical reasons also fell from 79% down to 46% [13]. In the United Kingdom, in 2013, hospital autopsies had declined to 0.69% of deaths on average [18]. A previous study in Northern Ireland showed rates declining from 21.6% to 7.9% from 1990-99 [6], while on follow-up, they were only performed in 0.46% of hospital deaths [18]. National data in the Netherlands showed a fall from 31.4% to 7.7% between 1977 and 2011 [46]. A national study in Australia found a decline from 21% in 1992-93 down to 12% in 2002-03 [12].

Literature from individual medical centers show more variable percentages but typically reflect the overall downward trend. Recent studies from major United States centers have reported rates of 12%-15% [30, 47, 48]. One hospital in Paris, France documented a decline from 15.4% in 1988 to 3.7% in 1997 [7]. A center in Zurich, Switzerland showed a delayed decline, with levels remaining around 94% from 1972-1992, but then decreasing to 54% by 2002 [15, 49]. A hospital in Australia reported a decrease from 47% in 1978 to 1.4% in 2015 [19]. Of note, a number of series have demonstrated markedly higher autopsy rates at large academic centers than in community hospitals [3, 48, 50–52]. This finding may explain some of the institutional rates that are higher than the national averages, and this trend should be kept in mind when considering autopsy rate data. A number of studies have also examined nursing homes and found autopsy rates as low as 1% or less; paired with the fact that the percentage of the overall population residing and dying in nursing homes has substantially increased over time, the low rate of autopsies in this particular setting has been found to contribute to the overall rate decline [5, 17].

Forensic, coroner, or medical-legal autopsy rates have not changed as dramatically as medical autopsy rates. Numerous studies from various locations demonstrate minimal to no decline in the rates of these autopsies [6, 10, 14, 46]. In some cases, medical-legal autopsy rates have been seen to increase, even as medical autopsies decreased [9, 53]. In other cases, while autopsies of all types decreased, the relative proportion of medical-legal autopsies increased [13]. In some places around the world, coroner autopsies are performed much more frequently than hospital autopsies. These differences in local practices must also be taken into account when considering autopsy rate data [18, 53].

Stratification of the above summary data reveals additional interesting trends. For instance, the autopsy rate varies dramatically by age. It has been observed that younger patients undergo autopsy at a much higher rate than older patients, peaking around the third decade and declining to very low rates by the end of the ninth decade of life [54, 55]. Davies et al. documented that adult autopsy rates are declining much more dramatically than those in infants and young children [12]. Neonatal autopsies are also declining in some centers [21]. It is therefore important to bear in mind that some studies include only adult autopsies [16, 56–58], some specifically exclude infants and stillborns [48, 59], and others include patients of all ages [12, 54]. Numerous studies have also documented gender differences, with men often undergoing autopsy at higher rates than women. The degree of gender difference is greater in some than others [5, 15-17, 48, 52, 57, 60–64], and some data do not reflect this trend [1, 51]. A prospective study noted that permission to perform an autopsy was more likely to be obtained from a female relative, which might partially account for this gender difference [65]. An Austrian group indicated that rates were falling more quickly in some regions of the country than others [14]. It has also been suggested that rates may decrease more dramatically among patients with particular medical conditions. For example, work from Switzerland found that autopsy rates among cancer patients dropped from 60% in 1980 to 7% in 2010, which they noted to be a faster and more dramatic decline than the country's overall autopsy rate [17]. Others, however, found similar rates between different causes of death [5]. Looking at only the overall rates does not provide the entire picture. Assessing specific reasons for declining rates among subgroups may be informative or help guide interventions.

In most places in the world, it is required for families to consent to a medical autopsy before it can be performed [2, 7]. Overall rate data do not capture whether families refuse autopsies or clinicians do not offer one. Either or both of these factors could contribute to the rate. Interestingly, available data addressing this issue are quite mixed. Burton and Underwood found in the United Kingdom that clinicians requested autopsy in only about 6% of cases, but that families agreed in 43% of these [10]. An American study from a similar time period found that requests were made 64% of the time, but permission was only granted in 31% [54]. In the Netherlands, it was found that autopsies were requested in up to 83% of deaths, but families agreed to autopsy in slightly under 19% of cases [56]. Strikingly similar rates were observed in Australia, with an 84% request rate and a 22% agreement rate [2]. In prospective intervention studies, significantly higher rates of requests and agreements have been attained, as will be explored later [65–69]. Which member of the health care team makes the request could also contribute to the request and agreement rates. Numerous papers highlight the fact that physicians are most often responsible for requesting autopsies [10, 56, 70, 71]. While house officers are sometimes the principal team members performing this task [10], attending and resident physicians may both make requests in other settings [56, 71]. McPhee et al. noted that requests by attending physicians were not more likely to be successful than those made by residents [71]. The reasons for these variable request and agreement rates are likely multifactorial and situation-specific. However, both clinician and family perception of the autopsy and approach to the decision process are likely principal factors and would benefit from deeper analysis. The opinions and dynamics informing this interaction, or lack of interaction, will be discussed further.

REASONS FOR FALLING AUTOPSY RATES

As discussed previously, successful completion of an autopsy typically requires a clinician making a request and a patient's family agreeing to an autopsy. Thus, physician and family attitudes may inform whether requests are made and whether they are accepted. Institutional policies and attitudes may also contribute to the request rate. Beliefs about autopsy are of course informed by culture and thus may differ based on location, religious beliefs, and other such factors. These cultural components may or may not be reflected in the available data, but should be kept in mind.

Clinician attitudes toward autopsy are shaped in part by medical school education. There is a broad range of medical student exposure to autopsy. In the United States, some programs offer autopsy experience during preclinical years, while others only expose students, if they elect to take dedicated pathology electives or fellowships [72–74]. One survey of United States pathology programs indicated that approximately 20% of medical students never have an opportunity to attend autopsies at all [72]. Medical students report a range of experiences and attitudes when surveyed directly. In general, they report that attending autopsies was a benefit to their education, contributing to understanding of anatomy, physiology, and clinical reasoning [74–76]. Unfortunately, students also regularly report negative emotional or visceral reactions to the autopsies [75, 76]. Students generally considered autopsies less useful for clinical purposes than for educational purposes and suggested they might be wasteful [75]. Students who have these experiences early in training may carry these impressions forward to instances when they need to request autopsies later in their careers. Alternative experiences, such as a virtual autopsy, may be able to provide the same level of relevant background information without provoking emotional responses. This lack of response may save students from short-term unpleasantness, but may make the experience less memorable in the long term [77].

Resident physicians are frequently tasked with requesting autopsies. Interestingly, numerous studies have highlighted that residents view autopsies positively based on their ability to reveal new information about patient cases and advance medical knowledge [47, 78, 79]. Despite these identified benefits, clinical residents only rarely attend autopsies [2, 72]. Residents also frequently note that they feel uncomfortable requesting autopsies. In some cases, this is attributed mainly to not knowing many details about the procedure or not having been trained in how to make such requests [80]. In other cases, requests are avoided due to either observed family distress or concerns about provoking distress [47, 79]. Interestingly, one study noted significant variability between individual residents in their rates of requesting autopsies [81]. Taken together, these data suggest that while attitudes are overall positive, dedicated training and increased efforts to make requests may substantially improve request rates.

Both attending and resident physicians frequently cite feelings of certainty about premortem diagnoses as a reason why autopsies are not necessary [56, 81]. In some cases, availability of newer diagnostic tools may contribute to clinicians' heightened diagnostic confidence [6, 82]; however, others found that this may not be the case [83]. Interestingly, a number of studies have found trends suggesting that clinicians can predict which autopsy cases will reveal novel diagnostic information. Such a trend would support making autopsy requests preferentially in cases of confusion or uncertainty; these trends did not typically achieve statistical significance when examined [51, 65, 84]. Furthermore, the rates of diagnostic discrepancy are sufficiently high, even in cases when clinicians are confident in diagnoses that this trend may not be clinically meaningful [51]. At least based upon available data, clinicians cannot justify deferring a request simply because they think they know the cause of death.

Fears of litigation are also frequently noted as a reason why clinicians hesitate to request autopsy. Wilkes and coworkers noted that concerns about legal action were the most frequent negative aspect of autopsy that resident physicians reported [78]. In contrast, Hooper and Geller noted a much smaller proportion of respondents feared litigation, and in fact, the majority did not think it was a contributor to falling autopsy rates [83]. One center with a dedicated bereavement and autopsy administrative staff noted a very low malpractice suit rate, attributed mainly to honest and delicate handling of such issues [85]. Bove and Iery in inspecting outcomes of 99 medical malpractice appeals cases found that autopsy findings most often helped defendants or were of secondary importance to other findings and concluded that fears of autopsy results are typically irrational [86].

Interestingly, pathologist attitudes about autopsy have received less objective coverage in the literature. On a more subjective basis, it has been suggested that many pathologists view autopsies as unpleasant and laborious tasks for which they are not properly compensated. They may also crave more interaction with their clinical colleagues in planning or discussing these endeavors [30]. Survey data support this latter point [87]. It is also clear that the majority of pathology faculty and residents consider the autopsy important for educational purposes [47, 72, 88]. Nevertheless, it has been suggested that autopsy requirements during pathology residency be eliminated to allow for more time in other areas of pathology, a viewpoint that has been controversial [89]. Proponents of the autopsy suggest that recognition of autopsy pathology as a formal subspecialty and appropriate recognition of these pathologists' academic contributions may help improve attitudes and opinions [47, 85, 90, 91].

Family attitudes about autopsy influence whether or not they agree to any requests that are made. General public perception of the autopsy is difficult to study. Some have approached such research through surveys, while others have examined popular media for autopsy-related content. These studies suggest that the public is reasonably well informed about the basic aspects of the procedure and some of its benefits [92–95]. Families may benefit from additional counseling about the appearance of the body after the procedure as well as its application to hospitalized patients. Respondents to one survey were much more familiar with autopsy used for suspicious or unattended deaths compared with hospital deaths [94]. The patient's own attitudes about autopsy, expressed prior to death, may occasionally inform the family's choices after death. Interestingly, families may decline autopsy due in part to concerns that the patient would not have wanted an autopsy [71]. However, several studies suggest that agreeing to one's own autopsy would be more favorable for some patients than agreeing to one for a family member [66, 95, 96]. This attitude was age-dependent and decreased in middle-aged compared to younger survey respondents [95]. It may be that more open dialogue among families would assuage concerns about unwanted postmortem procedures. Several additional concerns have been noted. Numerous studies have described family concerns about disfigurement or disrespectful handling of the body. In many cases, families feel that a loved one has "suffered enough" prior to death [47, 56, 71, 96]. Practical concerns such as delaying a funeral may also factor into the decision [71, 97]. For other families, religious beliefs significantly inform whether an autopsy may be performed or not [2, 56,

80, 98]. Family certainty about the cause of death may also be a factor [97]. Blokker et al. noted that a full half of refused requests were attributed to families' perceived certainty about the diagnosis. Clinicians reported these family reactions to the authors, which complicate interpretation of the data; nonetheless, the results are striking [56]. Conversely, Connell and colleagues in focusing on dementia in the elderly found that many would appreciate having a confirmation of the diagnosis of Alzheimer's disease [96]. Realistic discussions about premortem diagnostic confidence and the information that might be obtained in autopsy might help families make autopsy consent decisions.

Indeed, the nature of the discussion between clinicians and families often affects outcomes. In one survey of women who had experienced stillbirth or neonatal demise, one quarter could not recall being counseled about the benefits of autopsy [70]. Burton and coworkers found that the strength of the recommendation from a clinician was a key element in whether autopsy was agreed to or not [99]. Conversely, in a prospective intervention study that emphasized full and extensive discussions, not only were high agreement rates achieved, but 44% of families offered to donate organs for research or education even without being specifically asked to do so [100]. One group specifically examined the use of motivational interviewing and found that it improved rates of family agreement [101]. Thus, even though families may come into a discussion about autopsy with varying attitudes, having complete and detailed discussions may alleviate some of these concerns and increase rates of agreement.

Finally, various economic and policy factors, at the institutional, local, or national levels, may influence autopsy rates. From the early 1970s to today, many countries have experienced changes in policy regarding autopsy. In the United States, in 1971, the Joint Commission on the Accreditation of Hospitals eliminated a requirement that 20% of hospital deaths undergo autopsy in order to maintain accreditation [1]. This change removed a significant incentive to routinely request autopsies. One study performed in France attributed declining autopsy rates in part to changes in bioethics laws in 1994. An opt-out system, where an autopsy could be performed without permission unless it was specifically refused, became an opt-in system, where physicians were required to obtain permission in advance [7]. In Australia, it was observed that the decline from a 47% rate in 1979 to a 19% rate in 1989 coincided with passage of a similar law in 1982 [2]. In Switzerland, however, it was noted that rates had already been falling prior to passage of a similar law [17]. The authors of both of the prior studies fully acknowledge that these policies were neither primary nor principal factors contributing to declining autopsy rates [2, 7]. In Austria, where laws allowed autopsies to be performed without permission in any case deemed "interesting," they noted much higher overall autopsy rates [14]. This observation maintains the possibility that national policy plays a role in determining rates. One may also speculate that public attitudes about the autopsy may influence both the passage of these laws as well as the rates of agreement to perform an autopsy. The role of policy therefore remains convoluted and is unlikely to be fully unraveled.

Economic and fiscal issues are easier to quantify and easier to implicate in driving rates down. As pointed out in an analysis by Nemetz et al. the economic drivers of autopsy practice are simply not favorable [22]. On one hand, the costs of performing an autopsy are immediate, not inconsiderable, and are usually not reimbursed by insurance companies in the United States. As a result, the health care system must absorb the cost as part of the patient's care. On the other hand, the benefits of autopsies are less immediate and only sometimes quantifiable. Peace of mind or health benefits to family members are less economically pressing [22]. Interestingly, one survey of hospital administrators in Australia indicated that a vast majority of hospital administrators moderately to highly supported the importance of autopsy [12]. At least in some settings, it seems that the benefits outweigh the financial burden of performing autopsies.

PROBLEMS RESULTING FROM LOW AUTOPSY RATES

There are many benefits derived from autopsy. In-depth discussion of many of the clinical and scientific benefits are outside the scope of this chapter. Some benefits that arise on a case-by-case basis, such as helping individual families identify risks that may affect surviving family members, will not be considered here. However, a few key problems stem specifically from declining autopsy rates and merit discussion in this context.

One of the key benefits autopsy provides is the opportunity to confirm if premortem diagnoses were correct. Although the patient cannot benefit from these findings, clinicians can at least learn about any missed diagnoses and analyze what led to the error. As noted above, some clinicians cite increased diagnostic certainty as a reason for not requesting autopsies. However, diagnostic discrepancies detected by autopsies remain relatively high. A large number of studies have documented the prevalence of these errors [1, 4, 15-16, 48-52, 54, 57–59, 61–65, 84, 102–121]. By examining rates of errors detected at autopsy, Goldman et al. developed a classification system for diagnostic discrepancies [1]. Amendments have been suggested to this system in follow-up studies [50]. The authors defined two categories of major errors, defined as missed primary diagnoses. Class I errors occur when detection would have changed clinical management and may have led to patient survival. Class II errors would not have changed management, potentially because effective treatment is impossible or not available [1, 50]. Of note, some studies report major errors without stratifying into class I and class II, while others report these sub-categories [111]. Goldman et al. found virtually no changes in error rates between 1960, 1970, and 1980 [1]. However, a follow-up systematic review and meta-analysis demonstrated that major and, specifically, class I error rates have diminished over time [111]. The authors concluded that individual studies were likely underpowered to find a significant difference over time. Unfortunately, the study still detected an overall class I error rate of 9% among all autopsied deaths. It also projected that in the United States, most centers likely experience a class I error rate of 4.1-6.7% [111]. A number of additional investigations have also described declining error rates [15, 16, 49, 52]; however, others have clearly shown that discrepancies persist [57, 58]. Even if discrepancies have decreased, they have not gone down to zero. Furthermore, any given institution may experience a wide range of error rates. Without autopsy, an individual institution would have no idea what its discrepancy rate is, and diagnostic errors would likely go entirely undetected.

Studies of diagnostic discrepancy often explore the types of diagnoses that are missed clinically. Once again, the data are mixed in this respect. A classic, large study by Cameron and McGoogan cataloged conditions that were commonly over- or underdiagnosed clinically; myocardial infarction, pulmonary embolism, and cerebrovascular accident were all commonly both over- and underdiagnosed [105]. Acute abdominal conditions and neoplasms were frequently underdiagnosed. Several other investigators have revealed that discrepancies often prominently include myocardial infarction and pulmonary embolism [1, 4, 115, 118, 122]. More recent studies found that while these conditions remained among the most common diagnostic discrepancies; their numbers were falling, along with the overall discrepancy rate [52, 118]. Several studies have echoed the findings of unexpected neoplasms at autopsy as well [102, 113, 123, 124]. Additionally, the study by Goldman et al. indicated that the types of missed diagnoses may change over time [1]. Medical advances may create opportunities for certain entities to become more common. Their study noted, for example, the significant rise in opportunistic pathogens with the advent of immunosuppressive drugs. They also noted that certain diagnoses may change from class II to class I, as effective therapies become available for previously untreatable conditions [1].

Clinical setting may or may not impact diagnostic error rates. A number of studies have found significantly lower diagnostic error rates in university-affiliated hospitals than community hospitals [48, 50]. Within each hospital, however, error rates may not differ significantly. One study examined error rates between patients dying on a surgical ward, in a medical intensive care unit (ICU), and in affiliated nursing homes; the authors found no significant differences between discrepancies detected on autopsy [58]. An earlier study in the pediatric population found only non-statistically significant trends toward differences in the emergency department, ICU, and ward settings [108].

Discrepancies in the ICU setting have received particularly strong attention and have been reviewed extensively [34, 61–64, 107–110, 125-127]. Critically ill patients may have especially complex presentations or conditions that are difficult to sort out and diagnose. Interestingly, one systematic review found class I diagnostic discrepancy rates of 8%, quite similar to those of studies including broader clinical settings [126]. Some individual studies had much higher error rates [64, 107], while some were quite low [61, 127]. Blanco et al. specifically examined pediatric ICU patients undergoing special extracorporeal membrane oxygenation procedures and found especially high discrepancy rates, greater than 50%; however, the authors recognized that inability to transport these patients for diagnostic testing may have played a role [103]. Many of the missed diagnoses in the ICU setting were similar to those observed in other settings as well, including opportunistic fungal infections, myocardial infarctions, and unsuspected neoplasms [62, 63, 126]. The effect of the length of stay has also been examined, particularly in the ICU setting. One examination of this attributed many discrepancies to inadequate time available for evaluation prior to death [61]. Others, have noted either no differences in discrepancies depending on length of stay [63, 127] or in fact increasing discrepancies with increased length of stay [16, 128, 129]. It has been suggested that diagnostic momentum may promote diagnostic error in some of these situations, where early mistakes or assumptions are carried through a lengthy stay [50]. As with other topics discussed in this review, further interrogation of the reasons for differing rates in future studies would be especially informative.

Technological innovation has frequently been cited as a potential reason for decreasing autopsy rates. Clinicians often point to newer diagnostic tools, such as computed tomography scans, as a reason for increased diagnostic confidence [6, 82]. As discussed previously, clinician confidence is not a strong predictor of diagnostic discrepancies identified at autopsy. Similarly, newer technologies may not play a significant role in decreasing discrepancies. One study compared error rates in surgical, ICU, and nursing home patients also examined differences in diagnostic procedures [58]. As expected, the authors found significant differences in the extent of diagnostic workup between these three sites, but there were no differences in the extent of diagnostic workup between cases in which an error had been made versus those in which an error had not been made [58]. Combes and colleagues did not identify differences in the use of advanced diagnostic procedures between discrepant and non-discrepant cases [107]. In fact, several others have found that misleading findings on imaging contributed to diagnostic errors [1, 4, 48, 51]. A number of investigations present either mixed or conflicting findings. In one case, when the vast majority of patients had undergone imaging prior to death, it was determined that nearly one third of the causes of death could not have been seen on imaging [16]. Only half of the patients had the appropriate tests performed; 5.3% had imaging of the wrong anatomic location and 10% had an improper type of imaging performed. In another evaluation of pathology-radiology discrepancies, although over one quarter of cases were determined to be discrepant, only 3.3% were noted to be truly missed diagnoses of clinical significance; because of the limitations of both imaging and pathology, a small number of findings were determined to not have been detectable by one or the other [130]. Finally, one of the large independent studies that noted declining discrepancy rates also found significantly increasing numbers of diagnostic tests being performed [15]. Although the authors could only demonstrate a correlation, it is not out of the question that these diagnostic tests did play a partial causal role.

Features of data collection may impact some of these findings regarding diagnostic discrepancy. Several studies address the possibility of selection bias among cases chosen for autopsy. If clinicians are especially puzzled by a patient case, they might more aggressively request an autopsy [16]. As noted previously, clinicians have not been shown to accurately predict cases in which discrepancies are detected, which may partially address this concern [51, 84]. Of interest, one study that included a group of private autopsies, all of which were performed based on family-initiated request, found a strikingly high major error rate. Although this patient group also reflects a certain selection bias, it nonetheless raises the question as to whether families may be better at predicting discrepancy than clinicians [48]. As pointed out in the large systematic review referenced previously, meta analyses may be plagued by publication bias [111]. If studies that have striking or positive findings are more likely to be published than others, the data available in available publications may be skewed. Conversely, institutions may be hesitant to publish findings of especially large discrepancy rates. This possibility is more difficult to address but should be kept in mind when interpreting the discrepancy literature. Furthermore, determining the presence and type of a discrepancy during data collection may be imperfect. Whether this process is performed by a pathologist or by clinicians and pathologists together, or by looking at the autopsy request form versus by doing a thorough medical chart review, could influence the data [52, 111]. Of note, at least one study did check for inter-rater variability and found it to be minimal [50]. As with all studies, such factors related to data collection are difficult to control and care must be taken when interpreting individual studies.

Perhaps the most disturbing data problem is the revelation that discrepancy rate may be inversely related to autopsy rate. Although this issue has not been as widely addressed, several studies have documented that discrepancy rates tend to be lowest when autopsy rates are high [50, 111, 131]. One meta-analysis suggested that the trend was largely attributable to the presence of large academic centers in the data set that had higher autopsy rates but lower discrepancy rates [50]. Other studies have also questioned the legitimacy of this trend, and suggest that it may be due to an enrichment of difficult cases as overall rates fall [52]. As available research is conflicting, this finding would benefit from additional study and confirmation. We can only speculate about the reasons behind this trend. It may be that institutions that strive for high autopsy rates have a strong culture of quality improvement and use these autopsies as a tool for improving patient care. It is notable, for example, that the individual studies that detected declining error rates in fact had much higher overall autopsy rates than most other studies in the literature, even despite the rate of decline they reported [15, 49]. It may be that this institution had sufficiently high overall autopsy rates to effectively reduce diagnostic errors and allow the influence of technology or improved clinical reasoning to show through. Conversely, low autopsy rates may make it more difficult to control for selection bias or may highlight cases of misinterpreted testing or other major errors. Regardless of the reasons for this trend, its implications are clear: low institutional autopsy rates are correlated with higher institutional diagnostic error rates. Barring careful probing of the reasons behind this trend and/or efforts to increase the autopsy rates, many diagnostic errors are likely to remain undetected going forward.

Undetected errors have a number of concerning implications aside from quality improvement and patient safety. Especially in lieu of an autopsy, death certificates are typically completed based upon clinical data at time of death. A number of studies have demonstrated that large numbers of death certificates may be inaccurate due to lack of postmortem examination [60, 132–139]. Cameron and McGoogan found that, following autopsy, 27% of death certificates required reclassification of disease category under the international classification of diseases (ICD) code system [140]. A similar study in the United States found major errors in 29% of death certificates, and a further 26% had the right ICD category but the wrong specific diagnosis [133]. A study in the United Kingdom found that the sensitivity of the death certificate in predicting the actual cause of death was 0.47 [135]. Most of these studies reported differing rates of agreement based on disease process, with high rates of agreement for neurologic and neoplastic diseases but low rates for gastrointestinal and cardiovascular diseases [133–135]. Although these inaccuracies may or may not have significant impact, these data at minimum indicate that a large number of official documents may contain incorrect information.

Among the implications of death certificate inaccuracies is their impact on epidemiologic data. Population data regarding incidence and mortality rates for various illnesses are often based in part upon clinical data and death certificates. A number of studies have demonstrated that both the decline in autopsy rates and the issue of incorrect death certificates may impact statistics regarding cancer and cardiovascular disease [5, 136, 138, 139, 141]. In Switzerland, investigators did not detect a significant effect on cancer incidence rates due to the decline in autopsy rate; the authors noted declining rates of new cancer discovery at autopsy, while overall cancer incidence was steady or increasing [17]. Drawing on previous work, they suggest that improved diagnostic testing, prominently including the prostate-specific antigen test, may be improving premortem diagnosis [17, 142]. Since overall discrepancy rates tend to be lower for neoplastic processes than for cardiovascular disease, it is not entirely unexpected that cancer statistics might be impacted less than cardiovascular statistics [133–135]. Further investigation and an updated examination of this topic, especially with respect to cardiovascular statistics, would be beneficial.

INTERVENTIONS TO IMPROVE AUTOPSY RATE

Having described the global decline in autopsy rates and a few of the problems that result, we may thankfully describe a few interventions to address these issues. Some of these have yielded more promising results than others in preliminary investigations, but we will describe several that have proven to be major trends.

A few studies describe the elements of existing programs that had consistently high autopsy rates. In the United Kingdom, Champ et al. described holding death certificates in the morgue so that clinicians had to come and interact with the pathology staff in order to fill out a death certificate, with or without autopsy [143]. They concluded that this practice brought pathologists and clinicians closer together, encouraged clinician investment in autopsies and outcomes, and led to very high clinician attendance at the autopsy. Additionally, the pathology assistants in the morgue served an administrative role in certifying the deaths and coordinating meetings with families. This role would otherwise have been filled by administrative staff completely removed from the process [143]. Another American based evaluation reported a similar administrative arrangement with a dedicated decedent affairs staff associated with the department of pathology [85]. The authors described more effective risk management and litigation control with this structure. They also described extensive and open communication with clinicians, emphasizing timely result reporting. Finally, extensive academic involvement by the autopsy pathologists within the university setting improved their visibility, including required autopsy attendance by second-year medical students [85]. Clear themes emerge from these two studies, including fostering pathologist-clinician relationships and communication as well as a dedicated and well organized administrative structure.

Though the final autopsy rate achieved has varied considerably, all reported interventional studies of which we are aware have managed to increase autopsy rates substantially; most have approximately doubled pre-intervention autopsy rates [65, 67–69, 100]. Interestingly, most of these came out of departments of internal medicine rather than pathology. A number of common themes can be identified among the interventions. Virtually all of these involved increased efforts by clinicians to request autopsies for a greater percentage of hospital deaths. Of course, since most studies were clinician-driven, this feature was expected to a certain extent. Most interventions included specific training for residents about how to request an autopsy. There are also articles available in the literature offering instruction on how to do so [144]. One department also included education for social workers, hospital clergy, and administrators [67]. Of note, studies that tracked outcomes after the intervention ended found that rates fell sharply once the efforts were discontinued. This finding suggests that continuous effort is required to maintain autopsy rates, and may also suggest that lack of effort contributed greatly to the initial decrease in rates [69, 97].

A number of authors have investigated whether alternate postmortem procedures might be better accepted and more appropriate for modern medicine. Some have advocated for formal case discussions following each death; however, as has been described elsewhere, case discussions may miss diagnostic errors up to 85% of the time [15]. Others have suggested that involving certain selected specialists in these discussions may be more useful and could guide specified postmortem testing [145]. The use of postmortem imaging has also been extensively studied. It has been shown that procedures, such as whole-body magnetic resonance imaging, are able to detect a number of unexpected or confirmatory findings [146–152]. Radiologic approaches do miss some findings detectable on autopsy and cannot completely replace the procedure [130, 153]. Furthermore, imaging also carries substantial costs and is of limited availability in many hospitals [153]. While imaging may provide helpful information in some cases, it does not seem to be a suitable replacement for autopsy. Finally, some have advocated for minimally invasive or targeted autopsies [154–158]. In this approach, very limited tissue is taken, using techniques that preserve the external body to a greater degree than traditional autopsy, and may thus be more agreeable to families. These techniques obtain tissue of sufficient quality for histology or molecular testing [159]. Sampling misses diagnoses detected on autopsy, so this approach also cannot be used universally [157, 160]. In summary, there are a number of proposed alternatives to the traditional autopsy, but none fully addresses concerns with the typical approach and all seem to introduce additional drawbacks.

CONCLUSION

We have reviewed much of the available data regarding the global decline in autopsy rates. Since approximately 1970, rates of autopsies have been falling in countries around the world. Most major medical centers have also experienced falling rates. These changes have affected some patient populations more than others. In some places and some populations, the rates appear poised to drop to near zero. Multiple factors have been shown to contribute to this phenomenon. The attitudes of physicians as well as patients' families play a prominent role. Not only do surveys indicate a mutual discomfort with discussing autopsy, interventions that target this interaction significantly improve autopsy rates. Additionally, economic and policy factors at the institutional, local, and national levels may influence attitudes about the procedure, although policies are shaped by these attitudes as well. The autopsy offers numerous benefits, but key among these is the ability to detect diagnostic errors or resolve diagnostic dilemmas. When utilized properly, the autopsy provides opportunities for both learning and quality improvement. However, when rates are low, discrepancies go undetected and may increase, causes of death are recorded incorrectly, and important statistics may be inaccurate.

A number of interventions have successfully improved autopsy rates in some centers. By placing renewed emphasis on the procedure and its benefits, building strong relationships between clinicians and pathologists, and teaching physicians in training how to discuss autopsy with families, rates may be greatly improved.

REFERENCES

[1]   Goldman, L., Sayson, R., Robbins, S., Cohn, L. H., Bettmann, M., and Weisberg, M. (1983) The value of the autopsy in three medical eras. *N. Engl. J. Med.,* 308: 1000–5.

[2]   McKelvie, P. A. and Rode, J. (1992) Autopsy rate and a clinicopathological audit in an Australian metropolitan hospital - cause for concern? *Med. J. Aust.,* 156: 456–62.

[3]   Baker, P. B., Zarbo, R. J., and Howanitz, P. J. (1996) Quality assurance of autopsy face sheet reporting, final autopsy report turnaround time, and autopsy rates: A College of American Pathologists Q-Probes study of 10003 autopsies from 418 institutions. *Arch. Pathol. Lab. Med.,* 120: 1003–8.

[4]   Kirch, W. and Schafii, C. (1996) Misdiagnosis at a university hospital in 4 medical eras: report on 400 cases, *Medicine (Baltimore),* 75: 29-40.

[5]   Lindstrom, P., Janzon, L., and Sternby, N. H. (1997) Declining autopsy rate in Sweden: a study of causes and consequences in Malmö, Sweden, *J. Intern. Med.,* 242: 157–65.

[6]   Loughrey, M. B., McCluggage, W. G., and Toner, P. G. (2000). The declining autopsy rate and clinicians' attitudes. *Ulster Med. J.,* 69: 83–9.

[7]   Chariot, P., Witt, K., Pautot, V., Porcher, R., Thomas, G., Zafrani, E. S., and Lemaire, F. (2000). Declining autopsy rate in a French hospital. *Arch. Pathol. Lab. Med.,* 124: 739–45.

[8]   Sinard, J. H., and Blood, D. J. (2001). Quality improvement on an academic autopsy service. *Arch. Pathol. Lab. Med.,* 125: 237–45.

[9]   Wood, M. J., and Guha, A. K. (2001). Declining clinical autopsy rates versus increasing medicolegal autopsy rates in Halifax, Nova Scotia. *Arch. Pathol. Lab. Med.,* 125: 924–30.

[10] Burton, J. L. and Underwood, J. C. E. (2003). Necropsy practice after the "organ retention scandal": requests, performance, and tissue retention. *J. Clin. Pathol.,* 56: 537–41.

[11] Carr, U., Bowker, L., and Ball, R. Y. (2004). The slow death of the clinical post-mortem examination: implications for clinical audit, diagnostics and medical education, *Clin. Med.,* 4: 417–23.

[12] Davies, D. J., Graves, D. J., Landgren, A. J., Lawrence, C. H., Lipsett, J., MacGregor, D. P., and Sage, M. D., The Royal College of Pathologists of Australia Autopsy Working Party. (2004). The decline of the hospital autopsy: a safety and quality issue for healthcare in Australia. *Med. J. Aust.,* 180: 281–5.

[13] Hoyert, D. L. (2011). The changing profile of autopsied deaths in the United States, 1972 – 2007. *NCHS Data Brief,* 67: 1–8.

[14] Gaensbacher, S., Waldhoer, T., and Berzlanovich, A. (2012). The slow death of autopsies: a retrospective analysis of the autopsy prevalence rate in Austria from 1990 to 2009. *Eur. J. Epidemiol.,* 27: 577–80.

[15] Schwanda-Burger, S., Moch, H., Muntwyler, J., and Salomon, F. (2012). Diagnostic errors in the new millennium: a follow-up autopsy study, *Mod. Pathol.* 25: 777–83.

[16] Kuijpers, C. C. H. J., Fronczek, J., van de Goot, F. R. W., Niessen, H. W. M., van Diest, P. J., and Jiwa, M. (2014). The value of autopsies in the era of high-tech medicine: discrepant findings persist. *J. Clin. Pathol.,* 67: 512-9.

[17] Bieri, U., Moch, H., Dehler, S., Korol, D., and Rohrmann, S. (2015) Changes in autopsy rates among cancer patients and their impact on cancer statistics from a public health point of view: a longitudinal study from 1980 to 2010 with data from Cancer Registry Zurich. *Virchows Arch.,* 466: 637–43.

[18] Turnbull, A., Osborn, M., and Nicholas, N. (2015). Hospital autopsy: endangered or extinct? *J. Clin. Pathol.,* 68: 601-4.

[19] Raut, A., Andrici, J., Severino, A., and Gill, A. J. (2016). The death of the hospital autopsy in Australia? The hospital autopsy rate is declining dramatically. *Pathology,* 48: 645–9.

[20] Blokker, B. M., Weustink, A. C., Hunink, M. G. M., Oosterhuis, J. W., and Terry, J. (2017). Autopsy rates in the Netherlands: 35 years of decline. *PLoS One,* 12: e0178200.

[21] Brodlie, M., Laing, I. A., Keeling, J. W., and McKenzie, K. J. (2002). Ten years of neonatal autopsies in tertiary referral centre: retrospective study. *BMJ,* 324: 761–3.

[22] Nemetz, P. N., Ludwig, J., and Kurland, L. T. (1987). Assessing the autopsy., *Am. J. Pathol.,* 128: 362–79.

[23] Beljan, J. R., Bohigian, G. M., Estes, H. E., Friedlander, I. R., Kennedy, W. R., Moxley, J. H, Salva, P. S., et al. (1987). Autopsy: a comprehensive review of current issues. *JAMA,* 258: 364–9.

[24] Landefeld, C. S. and Goldman, L. (1989). The autopsy in clinical medicine. *Mayo Clin. Proc.,* 64: 1185–89.

[25] Charlton, R. (1994). Autopsy and medical education: a review. *J. R. Soc. Med.,* 87: 232–6 (1994).

[26] McPhee, S. J. (1996). Maximizing the benefits of autopsy for clinicians and families: what needs to be done. *Arch. Pathol. Lab. Med.,* 120: 743–8.

[27] McPhee, S. J. and Bottles, K. (1985). Autopsy: moribund art or vital science? *Am. J. Med.,* 78: 107–13.

[28] Lundberg, G. (1998). Low-tech autopsies in the era of high-tech medicine: continued value for quality assurance and patient safety. *JAMA,* 280: 1273–4.

[29] Khong, T. Y. (2002). Falling neonatal autopsy rates. *BMJ,* 324: 749–50.

[30] Dehner, L. P. (2010). The medical autopsy: past, present, and dubious future. *Mo. Med.,* 107: 94–100.

[31] van den Tweel, J. G. and Wittekind, C. (2016). The medical autopsy as quality assurance tool in clinical medicine: dreams and realities. *Virchows Arch.,* 468: 75–81.

[32]   Shojania, K. G. and Burton, E. C. (2008). The vanishing nonforensic autopsy. *N. Engl. J. Med.,* 358: 873–5.

[33]   Ayoub, T. and Chow, J. (2008). The conventional autopsy in modern medicine. *J. R. Soc. Med.*, 101: 177–81.

[34]   Wong, A., Osborn, M., and Waldmann, C. (2015). Autopsy and critical care. *J. Intensive Care Soc.,* 16: 278–81 (2015).

[35]   Turnbull, A., Martin, J., and Osborn, M. (2015). The death of autopsy?, *Lancet,* 386: 2141.

[36]   Bassat, Q., Castillo, P., Alonso, P. L., Ordi, J., and Menéndez, C. (2016). Resuscitating the dying autopsy. *PLoS Med.,* 13: e1001927.

[37]   Stempsey, W. E. (2016). The penetrating gaze and the decline of the autopsy. *AMA J. Ethics* 18: 833-8.

[38]   Hall, P. A. (2004). Do we really need a higher necropsy rate? *Lancet,* 354: 2004.

[39]   O'Grady, G. (2003). Death of the teaching autopsy. *BMJ,* 327: 803–4.

[40]   Geller, S. A. (2015). Who will do my autopsy? *Arch. Pathol. Lab. Med.,* 139: 578–80.

[41]   Liao, J. M. and Singh, H. (2013). Reviving the autopsy as a diagnostic error–reduction tool. *Lab Med.,* 44: 186–90.

[42]   Goldman, B. (2016). Reviving the hospital autopsy. *Arch. Pathol. Lab. Med.,* 140: 503–4.

[43]   Hamza, A. (2017). Declining rate of autopsies: implications for anatomic pathology residents. *Autopsy Case Reports,* 7: 1–2.

[44]   Burton, J. L. and Underwood, J. (2007). Clinical, educational, and epidemiological value of autopsy. *Lancet,* 369: 1471–80.

[45]   Sherman, F. T. (2008). Resuscitating the geriatric autopsy: advance directives may be the answer. *Geriatrics,* 63: 5, 26.

[46]   Blokker, B. M., Weustink, A. C., Hunink, M. G. M., and Oosterhuis, J. W. (2017). Autopsy rates in the Netherlands: 35 years of decline. *PLoS One* 12, e0178200.

[47]   Hull, M. J., Nazarian, R. M., Wheeler, A. E., Black-Schaffer, W. S., and Mark, E. J. (2007). Resident physician opinions on autopsy importance and procurement. *Hum. Pathol.,* 38, 342–50.

[48] Tavora, F., Crowder, C. D., Sun, C.-C., and Burke, A. P. (2008). Discrepancies between clinical and autopsy diagnoses: a comparison of university, community, and private autopsy practices. *Am. J. Clin. Pathol.,* 129: 102–9.

[49] Sonderegger-lseli, K., Burger, S., Muntwyler, J., and Salomon, F. (2000). Diagnostic errors in three medical eras: a necropsy study. *Lancet,* 355: 2027–31.

[50] Battle, R., Pathak, D., Humble, C. G., Key, C., Vanatta, P., Hill, R., and Anderson, R. (1987). Factors influencing discrepancies between premortem and postmortem diagnoses. *JAMA,* 258: 339–44.

[51] Landefeld, C. S., Chren, M.-M., Myers, A., Geller, R., Robbins, S., and Goldman, L. (1988). Diagnostic yield of the autopsy in a university hospital and a community hospital. *N. Engl. J. Med.,* 318: 1249–54.

[52] Wittschieber, D., Klauschen, F., Kimmritz, A.-C., von Winterfeld, M., Kamphues, C., Scholman, H.-J., Erbersdobler, A. et al. (2012). Who is at risk for diagnostic discrepancies? Comparison of pre- and postmortal diagnoses in 1800 patients of 3 medical decades in east and west Berlin. PLoS One, 7: e37460.

[53] Lunetta, P., Lounamaa, A., and Sihvonen, S. (2007). Surveillance of injury-related deaths: medicolegal autopsy rates and trends in Finland. *Inj. Prev.,* 13: 282–4.

[54] Sinard, J.H. (2001). Factors affecting autopsy rates, autopsy request rates, and autopsy findings at a large academic medical center, *Exp. Mol. Pathol.* 70, 333–343.

[55] Ahronheim, J., Bernholc, A., and Clark, W. (1983). Age trends in autopsy rates: striking decline in late life. *JAMA,* 250: 1182–6.

[56] Blokker, B. M., Weustink, A. C., Hunink, M. G. M., and Oosterhuis, J. W. (2016). Autopsy of adult patients deceased in an academic hospital: considerations of doctors and next-of-kin in the consent process. *PLoS One,* 11: e0163811.

[57] Marshall, H. S. and Milikowski, C. (2017). Comparison of clinical diagnoses and autopsy findings: six-year retrospective study. *Arch. Pathol. Lab. Med.,* 141: 1262–6.

[58] Scordi-Bello, I. A., Kalb, T. H., and Lento, P. A. (2010). Clinical setting and extent of premortem evaluation do not predict autopsy discrepancy rates, *Mod. Pathol.* 23: 1225-30.

[59] Stevanovic, G., Tucakovic, G., Dotlic, R., and Kanjuh, V. (1986). Correlation of clinical diagnosis with autopsy findings: a retrospective study of 2,145 consecutive autopsies. *Hum. Pathol.,* 17: 1225–30.

[60] Karwinski, B. and Hartveit, F. (1989). Death certification: increased clinical confidence in diagnosis and lack of interest in confirmation by necropsy is not justified. *J. Clin. Pathol.,* 42: 13-17.

[61] Fröhlich, S., Ryan, O., Murphy, N., McCauley, N., Crotty, T., and Ryan, D. (2014). Are autopsy findings still relevant to the management of critically ill patients in the modern era? *Crit. Care Med.,* 42: 336-43.

[62] Tejerina, E., Esteban, A., Fernández-Segoviano, P., Rodríguez-Barbero, J. M., Gordo, F., Frutos-Vivar, F., Aramburu, J., Algaba, A., Salcedo García, O. G., and Lorente, J. A. (2012). Clinical diagnoses and autopsy findings: discrepancies in critically ill patients. *Crit. Care Med.,* 40: 842–6.

[63] Tejerina, E. E., Padilla, R., Abril, E., Frutos-Vivar, F., Ballen, A., Rodríguez-Barbero, J. M., Lorente, J. A., and Esteban, A. (2018). Autopsy-detected diagnostic errors over time in the intensive care unit. *Hum. Pathol.,* 76: 85–90.

[64] Roosen, J., Frans, E., Wilmer, A., Knockaert, D. C., and Bobbaers, H. (2000). Comparison of premortem clinical diagnoses in critically ill patients and subsequent autopsy findings. *Mayo Clin. Proc.,* 75: 562–7.

[65] Cameron, H. M., McGoogan, E., and Watson, H. (1980). Necropsy: a yardstick for clinical diagnoses. *Br. Med. J.,* 281: 985–8.

[66] Forest, F., Duband, S., and Peoc'h, M. (2011). The attitudes of patients to their own autopsy: a misconception. *J. Clin. Pathol.,* 64: 1037.

[67] Smith, R. D. and Zumwalt, R. E. (1984). One department's experience with increasing the autopsy rate. *Arch. Pathol. Lab. Med.,* 108: 455–7.

[68] Clayton, S. A. and Sivak, S. L. (1992). Improving the autopsy rate at a university hospital. *Am. J. Med.,* 92: 423–6.

[69] Lugli, A., Anabitarte, M., and Beer, J. (1999). Effect of simple interventions on necropsy rate when active informed consent is required. *Lancet,* 354: 1391.

[70] Khong, T. Y. (1997). Improving perinatal autopsy rates: who is counseling bereaved parents for autopsy consent? *Birth* 24: 55–7.

[71] McPhee, S. J., Bottles, K., Lo, B., Saika, G., and Crommie, D. (1986). To redeem them from death: reactions of family members to autopsy. *Am. J. Med.,* 80: 665-71.

[72] Horowitz, R. E. and Naritoku, W. Y. (2007). The autopsy as a performance measure and teaching tool. *Hum. Pathol.,* 38: 688–95.

[73] Talmon, G. (2010). The use of autopsy in preclinical medical education: a survey of pathology educators. *Arch. Pathol. Lab. Med.,* 134: 1047–53.

[74] Tazelaar, H., Schneiderman, H., Yaremko, L., and Weinstein, R. (1987). Medical students' attitudes toward the autopsy as an educational tool. *J. Med. Educ.,* 62: 66–8.

[75] Benbow, E. W. (1990). Medical students' views on necropsies. *J. Clin. Pathol.,* 43: 969–76.

[76] Bamber, A. and Quince, T. (2015). The value of postmortem experience in undergraduate medical education: current perspectives. *Adv. Med. Educ. Pract.,* 6: 159–70.

[77] Talmon, G. A., Czarnecki, D., and Bernal, K. (2014). An effective virtual tool for exposing medical students to the postmortem examination. *Am. J. Clin. Pathol.,* 142: 594–600.

[78] Wilkes, M. S., Link, R. N., Jacobs, T. A., Fortin, A. H., and Felix, J. C. (1990). Attitudes of house officers toward the autopsy. *J. Gen. Intern. Med.,* 5: 122–5.

[79] Stolman, C., Castello, F., Yorio, M., and Mautone, S. (1994). Attitudes of pediatricians and pediatric residents toward obtaining permission for autopsy. *Arch. Pediatr. Adolesc. Med.,* 148: 843–7.

[80] Rosenbaum, G., Burns, J., Johnson, J., Mitchell, C., Robinson, M., and Truog, R. (2000). Autopsy consent practice at US teaching hospitals: results of a national survey. *Arch. Intern. Med.,* 160: 374–80.

[81] Hinchliffe, S. A., Godfrey, H. W., and Hind, C. R. K. (1994). Attitudes of junior medical staff to requesting permission for autopsy. *Postgrad. Med. J.,* 70: 292–4.

[82] Midelfart, J. and Aase, S. (1998). The value of autopsy from a clinical point of view. *APMIS,* 106: 693–8.

[83] Hooper, J. E. and Geller, S. A. (2007). Relevance of the autopsy as a medical tool: a large database of physician attitudes. *Arch. Pathol. Lab. Med.,* 131: 268–74.

[84] Bloor, M., Robertson, C., and Samphier, M. (1989). Occupational status variations in disagreements on the diagnosis of cause of death. *Hum. Pathol.,* 20: 144–8.

[85] Haque, A. K., Patterson, R. C., and Grafe, M. R. (1996). High autopsy rates at a university medical center: what has gone right? *Arch. Pathol. Lab. Med.,* 120: 727–32.

[86] Bove, K. E. and Iery, C. (2002). The role of the autopsy in medical malpractice cases, I: a review of 99 appeals court decisions. *Arch. Pathol. Lab. Med.,* 126: 1023–31.

[87] Anderson, R. E. and Hill, R. B. (1989). The current status of the autopsy in academic medical centers in the United States. *Am. J. Clin. Pathol.,* 92: S31–7.

[88] Hill, R. B. and Anderson, R. E. (1991). The uses and value of autopsy in medical education as seen by pathology educators. *Acad. Med.,* 66: 97-100.

[89] Davis, G. G., Winters, G. L., Fyfe, B. S., Hooper, J. E., Iezzoni, J. C., Johnson, R. L., Markwood, P. S., et al. (2018). Report and recommendations of the association of pathology chairs' autopsy working group. *Acad. Pathol.,* 5: 2374289518793988.

[90] van den Tweel, J. G. (2008). Autopsy pathology should become a recognised subspecialty. *Virchows Arch.,* 452: 585–7.

[91] Mrak, R. E., Parslow, T. G., and Ducatman, B. S. (2018). Benchmarking subspecialty practice in academic anatomic pathology: the 2017 association of pathology chairs survey. *Acad. Pathol.,* 5: 2374289518798556.

[92] Brown, H. G. (1984). Lay perceptions of autopsy. *Arch. Pathol. Lab. Med.,* 108: 446–8.

[93] Brown, H. G. (1990). Perceptions of the autopsy: Views from the lay public and program proposals. *Hum. Pathol.,* 21: 154–8.

[94] Start, R. D., Saul, C. A., Cotton, D. W. K., Mathers, N. J., and Underwood, J. C. E. (1995). Public perceptions of necropsy. *J. Clin. Pathol.,* 48: 497–500.

[95] Sanner, M. (1994). A comparison of public attitudes toward autopsy, organ donation, and anatomic dissection: a Swedish survey. *JAMA,* 271: 284-8.

[96] Connell, C. M., Avey, H., and Holmes, S. B. (1997). Attitudes about autopsy: implications for educational interventions. *Gerontologist,* 34: 665–73.

[97] Souza, V. L. and Rosner, F. (1997). Increasing autopsy rates at a public hospital. *J. Gen. Intern. Med.,* 12: 315–7.

[98] Gatrad, A. R. (1994). Muslim customs surrounding death, bereavement, postmortem examinations, and organ transplants. *BMJ.* 309: 521.

[99] Burton, E. C., Phillips, R. S., Covinsky, K. E., Sands, L. P., Goldman, L., Dawson, N. V., Connors Jr, A. F., and Landefeld, C. S. (2004). The relation of autopsy rate to physicians' beliefs and recommendations regarding autopsy. *Am. J. Med.,* 117: 255–61.

[100] Tsitsikas, D. Brothwell, M., Chin Aleong, J.-A., and Lister, A. T. (2011). The attitudes of relatives to autopsy: a misconception. *J. Clin. Pathol.,* 64: 412–4.

[101] Rosenberg, I., Gierer, B., Flury, R., Battegay, E., and Balmer, P. E. (2018). Motivational interviewing increases autopsy rates. *Swiss Med. Wkly.,* 148: w14679.

[102] Avgerinos, D. V. and Bjornsson, J. (2001). Malignant neoplasms: discordance between clinical diagnoses and autopsy findings in 3,118 cases. *APMIS,* 109: 774–80.

[103] Blanco, C., Steigman, C., Probst, N., Stroud, M., Bhutta, A. T., Dyamenahalli, U., Imamura, M., and Prodhan, P. (2014). Discrepancies between autopsy and clinical findings among patients requiring extracorporeal membrane oxygenator support. *ASAIO J.,* 60: 207-10.

[104] Burton, E. C., Troxclair, D. A., Newman, W. P. (1998). Autopsy diagnoses of malignant neoplasms: how often are clinical diagnoses incorrect? *JAMA,* 280: 1245–8.

[105] Cameron, H. M. and McGoogan, E. (1981). A prospective study of 1152 hospital autopsies: II. analysis of inaccuracies in clinical diagnoses and their significance. *J. Pathol.,* 133: 285–300.

[106] Pinto Carvalho, F. L., Cordeiro, J. A., and Cury, P. M. (2008). Clinical and pathological disagreement upon the cause of death in a teaching hospital: analysis of 100 autopsy cases in a prospective study. *Pathol. Int.,* 58: 568–71.

[107] Combes, A., Mokhtari, M., Couvelard, A., Trouillet, J., Baudot, J., Henin, D., Gibert, C., and Chastre, J. (2004). Clinical and autopsy diagnoses in the intensive care unit: a prospective study. *Arch. Intern. Med.,* 164: 389–92.

[108] Goldstein, B., Metlay, L., Cox, C., and Rubenstein, J. S. (1996). Association of pre mortem diagnosis and autopsy findings in pediatric intensive care unit versus emergency department versus ward patients. *Crit. Care Med.,* 24: 683-6.

[109] Pastores, S. M., Dulu, A., Voigt, L., Raoof, N., Alicea, M., and Halpern, N. A. (2007). Premortem clinical diagnoses and postmortem autopsy findings: discrepancies in critically ill cancer patients. *Crit. Care,* 11: R48.

[110] Perkins, G. D., McAuley, D. F., Davies, S., and Gao, F. (2003) Discrepancies between clinical and postmortem diagnoses in critically ill patients: an observational study. *Crit. Care,* 7, R129–32.

[111] Shojania, K. G., Burton, E. C., McDonald, K. M., and Goldman, L. (2003). Changes in rates of autopsy-detected diagnostic errors over time: a systematic review. *JAMA,* 289: 2849–56.

[112] Bombí, J. A., Ramírez, J., Solé, M., Grau, J. M., Chabas, E., Astudillo, E., Nicolás, J. M., and Balasch, J. (2003). Clinical and autopsy correlation evaluated in a university hospital in Spain (1991-2000). *Pathol. Res. Pract.,* 199: 9–14.

[113] Parajuli, S., Aneja, A., and Mukherjee, A. (2016). Undiagnosed fatal malignancy in adult autopsies: a 10-year retrospective study. *Hum. Pathol.,* 48: 32–6.

[114] Pelletier, L. L., Klutzow, F., and Lancaster, H. (1989). The autopsy: its role in the evaluation of patient care. *J. Gen. Intern. Med.,* 4: 300–3.

[115] Saad, R., Yamada, A. T., Da Rosa, F. H. F. P., Gutierrez, P. S., and Mansur, A. J. (2007). Comparison between clinical and autopsy diagnoses in a cardiology hospital. *Heart,* 93: 1414–9.

[116] Veress, B. and Alafuzoff, I. (1988). A retrospective analysis of clinical diagnoses and autopsy findings in 3,042 cases during two different time periods. *Hum. Pathol.,* 25: 140–5.

[117] Zarbo, R. J., Baker, P. B., and Howanitz, P. J. (1999). The autopsy as a performance measurement tool - diagnostic discrepancies and unresolved clinical questions: A College of American Pathologists Q- Probes study of 2479 autopsies from 248 institutions. *Arch. Pathol. Lab. Med.,* 123: 191–8.

[118] Thurnheer, R., Hoess, C., Doenecke, C., Moll, C., Muntwyler, J., and Krause, M. (2009). Diagnostic performance in a primary referral hospital assessed by autopsy: evolution over a ten-year period. *Eur. J. Intern. Med.,* 20: 784-7.

[119] Thurlbeck, W. M. (1981). Accuracy of clinical diagnosis in a Canadian teaching hospital. *Can. Med. Assoc. J.,* 125: 443–7.

[120] Gough, J. (1985). Correlation between clinical and autopsy diagnoses in a community hospital. *Can. Med. Assoc. J.,* 133: 420–2.

[121] Scottolini, A. G. and Weinstein, S. R. (1983). The autopsy in clinical quality control. *JAMA,* 250: 1192–4.

[122] Zarling, E. J., Sexton, H., and Milnor, P. (1983). Failure to diagnose acute myocardial infarction: the clinicopathologic experience at a large community hospital. *JAMA,* 250: 1177–81.

[123] Karwinski, B., Svendsen, E., and Hartveit, F. (1990). Clinically undiagnosed malignant tumours found at autopsy. *APMIS,* 98: 496–500.

[124] Podduturi, V., Guileyardo, J. M., Soto, L. R., and Krause, J. R. (2015). A case series of clinically undiagnosed hematopoietic neoplasms discovered at autopsy. *Am. J. Clin. Pathol.,* 143: 854–60.

[125] De Vlieger, G. Y. A., Mahieu, E. M. J. L., and Meersseman, W. (2010). Clinical review: what is the role for autopsy in the ICU? *Crit. Care,* 14: 221.

[126] Winters, B., Custer, J., Galvagno, S. M., Colantuoni, E., Kapoor, S. G., Lee, H., Goode, V., et al. Diagnostic errors in the intensive care unit: a systematic review of autopsy studies. *BMJ Qual. Saf.,* 21: 894-902.

[127] Nadrous, H. F., Afessa, B., Pfeifer, E. A., and Peters, S. G. (2003). The role of autopsy in the intensive care unit. *Mayo Clin. Proc.,* 78: 947–50.

[128] Mort, T. C. and Yeston, N. S. (1999). The relationship of pre mortem diagnoses and post mortem findings in a surgical intensive care unit. *Crit. Care Med.,* 27: 299–303.

[129] Maris, C., Martin, B., Creteur, J., Remmelink, M., Piagnerelli, M., Salmon, I., Vincent, J. L., and Demetter, P. (2007). Comparison of clinical and post-mortem findings in intensive care unit patients. *Virchows Arch.,* 450: 329–33.

[130] Murken, D. R., Ding, M., Branstetter, B. F., and Nichols, L. (2012). Autopsy as a quality control measure for radiology, and vice versa. *Am. J. Roentgenol.,* 199: 394–401.

[131] Shojania, K. G., Burton, E. C., McDonald, K. M., and Goldman, L. (2005). Overestimation of clinical diagnostic performance caused by low necropsy rates. *Qual. Saf. Heal. Care,* 14: 408-13.

[132] Schottenfeld, D., Eaton, M., Sommers, S. C., Alonso, D. R., and Wilkinson, C. (1982). The autopsy as a measure of accuracy of the death certificate. *Bull. N. Y. Acad. Med.,* 58: 778–94.

[133] Kircher, T., Nelson, J., and Burdo, H. (1985). The autopsy as a measure of accuracy of the death certificate. *N. Engl. J. Med.,* 313: 1263–9.

[134] Maclaine, G. D., Macarthur, E. B., and Heathcote, C. R. (1992). A comparison of death certificates and autopsies in the Australian Capital Territory. *Med. J. Aust.,* 156: 462–8.

[135] Sington, J. and Cottrell, B. (2002). Analysis of the sensitivity of death certificates in 440 hospital deaths: a comparison with necropsy findings. *J. Clin. Pathol.* 55: 499–502.

[136] Smith, C. J., Scott, S. M., and Wagner, B. M. (1998). The necessary role of the autopsy in cardiovascular epidemiology. *Hum. Pathol.,* 29: 1469–79.

[137] McKelvie, P. A. (1993). Medical certification of causes of death in an Australian metropolitan hospital. *Med. J. Aust.,* 158: 816–21.

[138] Kircher, T. (1990). The autopsy and vital statistics. *Hum. Pathol.,* 21 166–73.

[139] Hoel, D. G., Ron, E., Carter, R., and Mabuchi, K. (1993). Influence of death certificate errors on cancer mortality trends. *J. Natl. Cancer Inst.,* 85: 1063–8.

[140] Cameron, H. M. and McGoogan, E. (1981). A prospective study of 1152 hospital autopsies: I. inaccuracies in death certification. *J. Pathol.,* 133: 273–83.

[141] Burnand, B. and Feinstein, A. R. (1992). The role of diagnostic inconsistency in changing rates of occurrence for coronary heart disease. *J. Clin. Epidemiol.,* 45: 929–40.

[142] Konety, B. R., Bird, V. Y., Deorah, S., and Dahmoush, L. (2005). Comparison of the incidence of latent prostate cancer detected at autopsy before and after the prostate specific antigen era. *J. Urol.,* 174: 1785–8.

[143] Champ, C., Tyler, X., Andrews, P. S., and Coghill, S. B. (1992). Improve your hospital autopsy rate to 40–50 per cent, a tale of two towns. *J. Pathol.,* 166: 405-7.

[144] Schneiderman, H. and Gruhn, J. (1985). How—and why—to request an autopsy. *Postgrad. Med.,* 77: 153–64.

[145] Laposata, M. (2017). A new kind of autopsy for 21st century medicine. *Arch. Pathol. Lab. Med.,* 141: 887–8.

[146] Wichmann, D., Obbelode, F., Vogel, H., Hoepker, W., Nierhaus, A., Braune, S., Sauter, G., Pueschel, K., and Kluge, S. (2012). Virtual autopsy as an alternative to traditional medical autopsy in the intensive care unit: a prospective cohort study. *Ann. Intern. Med.,* 156: 123–30.

[147] Patriquin, L., Kassarjian, A., O'Brien, M., Andry, C., and Eustace, S. (2001). Postmortem whole-body magnetic resonance imaging as an adjunct to autopsy: Preliminary clinical experience. *J. Magn. Reson. Imaging,* 13: 277–87.

[148] Roberts, I. S. D., Benamore, R. E., Benbow, E. W., Lee, S. H., Harris, J. N., Jackson, A., Mallett, S., et al. (2012). Post-mortem imaging as an alternative to autopsy in the diagnosis of adult deaths: a validation study. *Lancet,* 379: 136–42.

[149] Scholing, M., Saltzherr, T. P., Fung Kon Jin, P. H. P., Ponsen, K. J., Reitsma, J. B., Lameris, J. S., and Goslings, J. C. (2009). The value of postmortem computed tomography as an alternative for autopsy in trauma victims: a systematic review. *Eur. Radiol.,* 19: 2333–41.

[150] Thayyil, S., Chandrasekaran, M., Chitty, L. S., Wade, A., Skordis-Worrall, J., Bennett-Britton, I., Cohen, M., et al. (2010). Diagnostic accuracy of post-mortem magnetic resonance imaging in fetuses, children and adults: a systematic review. *Eur. J. Radiol.,* 75: e142–8.

[151] Thayyil, S., Sebire, N. J., Chitty, L. S., Wade, A., Chong, W. K., Olsen, O., Gunny, R. S. et al. (2013). Post-mortem MRI versus conventional autopsy in fetuses and children: a prospective validation study. *Lancet,* 382: 223–33.

[152] Westphal, S. E., Apitzsch, J., Penzkofer, T., Mahnken, A. H., Knüchel, R. (2012). Virtual CT autopsy in clinical pathology: feasibility in clinical autopsies. *Virchows Arch.,* 461: 211–9.

[153] Burton, E. C. and Mossa-Basha, M. (2012). To image or to autopsy? *Ann. Intern. Med.,* 156: 158–9.

[154] Carter, R. L. (1987). The role of limited, symptom-directed autopsies in terminal malignant disease. *Palliat. Med.,* 1: 31–36.

[155] Aghayev, E., Thali, M. J., Sonnenschein, M., Jackowski, C., Dirnhofer, D., and Vock, P. (2007). Post-mortem tissue sampling using computed tomography guidance. *Forensic Sci. Int.,* 166: 199–203.

[156] Weustink, A. C., Hunink, M. G. M., van Dijke, C. F., Renken, N. S., Krestin, G. P., and Oosterhuis, J. W. (2009). Minimally invasive autopsy: an alternative to conventional autopsy? *Radiology,* 250: 897–904.

[157] Foroudi, F., Cheung, K., and Duflou, J. (1995). A comparison of the needle biopsy post mortem with the conventional autopsy. *Pathology,* 27: 79–82.

[158] Huston, B. M., Malouf, N. N., and Azar, H. A. (1996). Percutaneous needle autopsy sampling. *Mod. Pathol.,* 9: 1101–7.

[159] van der Linden, A., Blokker, B. M., Kap, M., Weustink, A. C., Riegman, P. H. J., and Oosterhuis, J. W. (2014). Post-mortem tissue biopsies obtained at minimally invasive autopsy: an RNA-quality analysis. *PLoS One,* 9: e115675.

[160] Breeze, A. C. G., Jessop, F. A., Whitehead, A. L., Set, P. A. K., Berman, L., Hackett, G. A., and Lees, C. C. (2008). Feasibility of percutaneous organ biopsy as part of a minimally invasive perinatal autopsy. *Virchows Arch.,* 452: 201–7.

In: A Closer Look at Autopsies
Editor: Fernando Robertson

ISBN: 978-1-53617-178-5
© 2020 Nova Science Publishers, Inc.

Chapter 6

THE CONTINUING RELEVANCE OF AUTOPSIES: THE ROLE OF AUTOPSIES TODAY

Diane M. Libert and Richard Prayson, MD*

Cleveland Clinic Lerner College of Medicine
and Department of Anatomic Pathology,
Cleveland Clinic, Cleveland, OH, US

ABSTRACT

Autopsies have been performed for centuries and historically have served a variety of purposes. In more recent years, autopsy rates have significantly declined and some have argued that the autopsy has become somewhat obsolete given advances in technology and medicine. This article will review the purposes of performing autopsies and their continued relevancy. At a societal level, autopsies play a crucial role in public health and the justice system. They are necessary in understanding the causes and course of epidemic outbreaks and recognizing the emergence of new diseases. In the forensic area, autopsies are performed to explain the cause, mechanism, and manner of death. At an individual level, autopsies allow for a more complete understanding of a patient's

---

* Corresponding Author's Email: praysor@ccf.org.

disease course which may not have been clear while the patient was alive. This can provide great services to both medical teams and family members of the deceased. Even with advances in medicine, autopsies still uncover missed diagnoses. Much of what we know about many diseases today is the result of autopsies, and in fact, many diseases were first discovered and described at autopsy. Furthermore, autopsies provide a vehicle for ensuring quality care by providing information needed to develop safer medical practices, procedures, and instruments. These examinations can also help families both by bringing closure to the loss of a loved one and potentially uncovering familial or genetic diseases.

1. COMMON REASONS FOR PERFORMING AUTOPSIES

After World War II, approximately 50% of hospital deaths were sent to autopsy [1]. Since then, the autopsy rate has declined and averages at less than 10% today [2]. From 1972 to 2007, the ailments of those most commonly autopsied have changed. The autopsy rate for deaths from disease fell from 16.9% to 4.3% and that for external causes increased from 43.6% to 55.4% [3]. In 2007, only one of the top 10 most common reasons for autopsy (pregnancy, childbirth, and puerperium) was related to health or disease; the rest were due to external causes. Specifically, the top 10 most commonly autopsied cases were assault, legal intervention, events of undetermined intent, accidental poisoning, drowning and submersion, discharge of firearms, or exposure to smoke/fire, followed by suicide by other/unspecified means, pregnancy/childbirth/puerperium, and transport accidents. The age distribution of those autopsied has also shifted. In 1972, 37% of all decedents autopsied were aged 64 years or older, and this fell to 17% in 2007. Conversely, in 1972, those in the 35-64 and 1-34 year-old age groups comprised 41% and 15%, and these percentages rose to 54% and 24%, respectively.

Despite these changing indications, autopsy remains an important technique for many different reasons. A recent statement by the American Society of Clinical Pathology (ASCP) on the purposes of autopsy summarizes pathologist's point of view on this topic and lists the purposes as follows [4]:

1) Quality assurance of medical diagnostics and service
2) A reservoir of tissues and organs for transplantation and research
3) Public education
4) Development of accurate mortality statistics
5) Early identification of environmental, infectious, and occupational hazards to health
6) Information documentation for future legal, financial, and medical evaluation
7) Evaluation of new forms of therapy and new diagnostic modalities
8) Continuing education of physicians

2. PUBLIC HEALTH

Autopsies provide information that has wide-reaching public health implications including surveillance of infectious disease epidemics, environmental exposures, and preventative care.

The medical community needs to be constantly vigilant and quickly react to threats from infectious epidemics. In the unfortunate event of a disease with a high mortality rate, autopsies can provide critical information about the cause and course of disease. During the outbreak of severe acute respiratory syndrome (SARS) in 2003, 14 autopsies performed during the initial outbreak in Singapore led to the identification of the coronavirus as the cause of infection, as well as several of its clinical manifestations such as diffuse alveolar damage and pulmonary thromboemboli [5]. This information acquired early in the course of the outbreak provided clinicians with understanding critical to identifying this disease and anticipating its course.

Autopsies not only provide information important in identifying infectious epidemics in real time, they can also facilitate understanding of disease outbreaks in the past. For example, frozen tissue samples kept from the disastrous 1918 influenza epidemic were sequenced to learn more about the adaptation of this virus to humans [6]. Without these autopsy specimens, acquiring this knowledge would not have been possible.

In addition to providing knowledge necessary to treating victims of infectious agents, autopsies can lead to recognition of the health effects brought about by environmental exposures. Asbestos, which was manufactured and widely used for building and road materials in the early 20th century, was found to cause lung cancer and mesothelioma, a health risk which is now widely known and has led to a great reduction in its use. This discovery was critically expounded upon at autopsy [7, 8]. Another example is the discovery that polyvinyl chloride (PVC) exposure leads to the development of angiosarcoma; it was the findings on autopsy which alerted the treating clinicians to this risk factor [9]. This recognition led to the United States Occupational Safety and Health Administration proposing a 500-fold reduction in the occupational exposure standard for PVC in 1974 [10].

Autopsies have provided us with invaluable information to inform different types of preventative care from vehicle safety to health preventative measures. Cadavers have played an important role in biomechanical research. Important uses of cadavers in such a manner include duplicating injury-producing impacts in a controlled environment, understanding the mechanical response of body regions and organs to impact loading, understanding the mechanisms of injury, and designing anthropomorphic test devices (ATDs) and mathematical models [11].

Preventative care measures that target common causes of morbidity and mortality, are often identified based on death statistics. In America, death statistics are based on information collected from death certificates. Death certificates, which must be filled out by the attending physician within 48 hours of death, list the "more likely than not" cause of death [12]. Autopsies are not required to complete the death certificate, but several studies point to the fact that more information from autopsies would provide a more complete picture of the common causes of death. According to one study of 223 decedents who underwent autopsy within one community hospital, the death certificate missed acute myocardial infarction (MI) in 25 of 52 autopsy-proven cases and erroneously asserted the presence of acute MI in 9 out of 36 cases, underscoring the importance of correcting death certificates and providing evidence to support that increased autopsy numbers would improve the accuracy of vital statistics [13].

Autopsy studies both clarify causes of death and identify areas for intervention beforehand. One example is the findings of atherosclerotic changes in United States service members in the second and third decade of life, well before signs of ischemic heart disease [14]. The Bogalusa Heart Study characterized the presence and prevalence of atherosclerosis in the aorta and coronary arteries of young patients, aged 2-39 years old, as well as factors associated with greater atherosclerosis such as increased age, body mass index, blood pressure, and serum total and low-density lipoprotein cholesterol [15]. These works helped highlight the importance of early awareness and treatment for cardiovascular disease prevention.

Valuable information regarding public health is obtained through autopsies, which provide actionable clinical knowledge regarding both immediate factors such as infections and environmental exposures, and long-term lifestyle interventions such as vehicle safety and cardiovascular disease prevention.

3. FORENSICS

Forensic autopsies are performed to determine the cause of death and collect evidence that may be used in the prosecution of those alleged to be responsible. They are especially important in cases of violent and unexpected death involving social and legal issues. Medical examiners are forensic pathologists who perform these autopsies and often play an important role in piecing together the circumstances of the crime in question. Widely-known examples include Dr. Michael Baden, who was able to characterize bullet patterns when he examined Michael Brown, an 18-year-old African American shot by a white police officer in Ferguson, Missouri in 2014 [16]. Dr. Cyril Wecht, who examined John F. Kennedy after his assassination in 1963, shed light on evidence that the fatal shot of the late President was likely the one which entered in the back of the head [17]. Forensic pathology involves macropathology, radiological study, and laboratory investigation including microbiology, serology, and immunohistochemistry. Molecular pathology involves the use of genetic studies including the decedent's background gene expression as well as dynamic changes that may have occurred around death and subsequent metabolic deterioration [18]. Each of these techniques assists the investigator in determining the exact circumstances of death and in clarifying the role of any incidental findings on investigation.

4. MEDICAL CARE AND QUALITY CONTROL

Autopsies play an important role in medical care and quality control. In some instances, autopsy is critical for diagnosing the patient's cause of death and other conditions that may be important for the treating clinician or surviving family members to know (such as genetic conditions). Alzheimer's disease, can only by definitively diagnosed at autopsy, despite the wide availability of advanced imaging techniques such as magnetic resonance imaging and computed tomography. Autopsies also play an important role in understanding the causes of fetal death. Fetal autopsies allowed for the first characterization of congenital malformations [19]. In one study, autopsy was able to characterize over two-thirds of fetal deaths as noninfectious, placenta-related or infectious [20]. In the case of the unfortunate event of fetal death, autopsy is critical to informing both the physician and the family of the cause of death and bringing closure to the situation.

One of the reasons cited for the decline in autopsy rates in the last few decades is the fact that the diagnostic methods used before death have improved. This notion was investigated in a systematic review of 53 autopsy series between 1966 and 2002, which found a median major error (defined as a clinically missed diagnosis involving a primary cause of death) rate of 23.5% and class I error (using the Goldman criteria, where class I is defined as an error likely to have affected patient outcome) of 9.0% [21]. According to this study, both major and class I error rates declined through the decades, but the authors estimate that a contemporary

American hospital could observe a major error rate of 8.4-24.4% and a class I error rate of 4.1-6.7%, depending on the percentage of deaths autopsied [21]. Recognizing these discrepancies can inform patient care before death. For example, in a retrospective review of 658 cancer deaths in an Intensive Care Unit (ICU) from 1999-2005, 13% were autopsied, revealing a major missed diagnosis rate of 26% and a class I error rate of 54% [22]. Opportunistic infections and cardiac complications comprised most of these class I errors, which highlighted the need for clinicians to monitor these in critically ill cancer patients. Another review of 31 studies including 5863 autopsies from ICU deaths found that 28% of autopsies had at least one misdiagnosis with 8% identifying a class I error, with pulmonary embolism, myocardial infarction, pneumonia, and Aspergillosis comprising most of the class I errors [23].

In addition to informing the medical conditions to anticipate in hospitalized patients, autopsies also provide important information about medical equipment used today. A study on the post-mortem analysis of pacemakers led to the observation that patients with pacemakers need to be monitored very closely. For example, 71% of those who died had consulted a physician within 10 days of death for various reasons and that the cause and manner of death was associated with the pacemaker in up to 50% of the cases [24].

Procedures can also be evaluated by autopsy studies, especially those that are performed in emergency situations and are otherwise difficult to study. Examples include a study that assessed the performance of resuscitative thoracotomy and the utility of resuscitative endovascular balloon occlusion of the aorta (REBOA) [25, 26]. Each of these studies helps form and refine guidelines for the management of emergency situations. Complications of tube thoracostomy, such as lung perforation, have also explored through autopsy [27, 28].

Autopsies provide final diagnoses for patients, inform clinical practice for future patients before death, and demonstrate the effectiveness and consequences of medical equipment use and procedures on patients.

5. RESEARCH AND EDUCATION

Many conditions are only fully discovered and described at autopsy, and post-mortem procedures and dissection of cadavers are important teaching tools in medical education.

Throughout the years, autopsies have shed light on both the diagnoses themselves and the progression of diseases such as cancer as well as medication side effects. One historic example is the appendix as the source of variously named "peritonitis, generalized inflammation of the bowel, typhlitis, etc" which was generally fatal until Dr. Fitz, a pathologist in Boston, clarified its etiology [29]. Other diseases discovered or critically explained through autopsy involve those from every organ system and run the gamut from spongiform encephalopathy and congenital heart deformities to complications of diabetes mellitus [19]. Recently, research drawn from autopsy study has emphasized that in the era of prostate specific antigen (PSA) screening, overall incident prostate cancer is mainly indolent; among 6024 men aged 70-79 years in one study, 36% of Caucasians and 51% of African Americans had a prostate tumor [30]. This knowledge saves many men from painful and unnecessary interventions. Another fairly recent study similarly examined the incidence of ovarian cancer at autopsy [31].

Findings at autopsy have also directly informed clinical management. Post-mortem research and observations identified the increasing incidence of invasive fungal disease in immunocompromised patients, alerting treating clinicians to this issue for future patients [32]. 75% of the invasive fungal infections in one study were not identified until autopsy [33].

Side effects of therapies continue to be discovered and characterized through autopsy findings. Aplastic anemia and other cytopenias as a complication of drug therapies were discovered in this manner [19]. Additionally, the effects of radiation on the heart were clarified through autopsy studies [34, 35].

Though an ancient practice, autopsy study also lends itself to novel research. Molecular testing of one decedent during autopsy of an 18-year-old female who died suddenly revealed a novel mutation in the long QT syndrome type II gene KCNH2. Targeted testing in the family revealed that the mutation arose de novo, eliminating the need for annual cardiac follow-up and a costly genetic workout in the surviving family members [36]. There have been several other studies on the utility of performing a cardiac channel molecular autopsy in incidents of sudden unexplained death [37, 38].

Much of the early knowledge of anatomy comes from information gained from autopsy, and it continues to inform us about the human body. More specific information, such as the fact that pleuroperitoneal blebs occur less frequently in the left hemidiaphragm, as it seems to be thicker and more muscular, was discovered with autopsies [39]. A recent autopsy study focused on elucidating the anatomy of the posterior tibial artery [40].

In addition to uncovering new medical knowledge and side effects of medical treatments, post-mortem examinations can play an important role in educating medical students [41, 42]. Due to declining autopsy rates and less-favorable media treatment of autopsies, these are likely underused in medical education [42]. Autopsies serve various purposes during medical education including exposing students to the problem-based approach used by pathologists during the procedure, teaching macroscopic pathology and skills in clinical-pathological correlation as well as the shortcomings of medicine, medical ethics, and medical law. Opportunities to practice and witness the effects of invasive medical procedures are also available during autopsy.

The role of autopsies in research and education is multifaceted and valuable. Post-mortem studies provide material for the identification of new diseases and the progression of known diseases as well as side effects of drug treatments and procedures. In medical education, autopsies confer both knowledge of anatomy and exposure to the field of pathology and more profound concepts such as medical ethics and the eventual fallibility of medicine.

6. CLOSURE FOR FAMILIES

Knowledge of the common reasons that families request autopsies will likely help increase the frequency of physician's initiating discussions of autopsies with patient families and improving physician comfort levels. Attitudes toward autopsy in family members from 102 patient deaths were studied, including 62 family members from patients who had undergone autopsy [43]. Commonly cited reasons for wanting an autopsy performed included advancement of medical knowledge (76%), uncertainty about the cause of death (53%), recommendations of the physician (50%), and surviving family member wishes (35%). Less frequently listed reasons included organ donation (13%) and wishes of the deceased (11%). 68% of family members of those who underwent autopsy considered the autopsy moderately or extremely beneficial, and the most important benefits cited were advancement of medical knowledge (74%), comfort in knowing the cause of death (41%) and reassurance that appropriate care was given (34%). Another small survey of family members of a decedent that underwent autopsy helped to clarify the important factors for the family which helped in the grief process, namely reassurance that they had not overlooked important symptoms in the deceased [44]. In a survey of parents who consented to late fetal and neonatal autopsy, common reasons cited included the autopsy had helped to explain what happened; it helped to plan future pregnancies; and it helped families to come to terms with what had happened [45].

CONCLUSION

Autopsy rates have decreased in recent decades, but they still have vital roles in public health, the justice system, patient care, research, and education today. Post-mortem observations inform clinicians of conditions to monitor in patients before death, including chronic illnesses, co-morbid diseases, and more. Though data from death certificates comprise mortality statistics, the most definite method at the clinician's disposal to determine the underlying and immediate causes of death is the autopsy. Post-mortem exams performed for forensics can provide knowledge of the circumstances surrounding a patient's death that can be useful for legal proceedings. Research gained from autopsies provides knowledge on everything from disease progression and epidemiology, to procedures and interventions, to vehicle safety. Medical students have always learned a great deal from autopsies and this is still true today. Lastly, autopsies can provide family members and loved ones with closure regarding cause of death and gratification that the procedure helps to advance medical knowledge.

REFERENCES

[1]   Roberts, W. C. (1978). The autopsy: its decline and a suggestion for its revival. *N. Engl. J. Med.* 299, 332–338.

[2]   Levy, B. (2015). Informatics and autopsy pathology. *Surg. Pathol. Clin.* 8, 159–174.

[3]   Hoyert, D. L. (2011). The changing profile of autopsied deaths in the United States, 1972-2007. *NCHS Data Brief.*

[4]   *The American Society for Clinical Pathology Policy Statement: Autopsy (Policy Number 91–0)*, American Society for Clinical Pathology:

[5]   Chong, P. Y., Chui, P., Ling A. E., Franks, T. J., Tai, D. Y. H., Leo Y. S., et al. (2004). Analysis of deaths during the Severe Acute Respiratory Syndrome (SARS) epidemic in Singapore: challenges in determining a SARS diagnosis. *Arch. Pathol. Lab. Med.* 128, 195–204.

[6]   Taubenberger, J. K., Reid, A. H., Lourens, R. M., Wang, R., Jin, G., Fanning, T. G. (2005). Characterization of the 1918 influenza virus polymerase genes. *Nature* 437, 889–893.

[7]   Mossman, B. T. and Gee, J. B .L. (1989). Asbestos-related diseases. *N. Engl. J. Med.* 320, 1721–1730.

[8] Jones, J. S., Pooley, F. D., Clark, N. J., Owen, W. G., Roberts, G. H., Smith, P. G., et al. (1980). The pathology and mineral content of lungs in cases of mesothelioma in the United Kingdom in 1976. *IARC Sci. Publ.* 187-199.

[9] Creech, J. L. J. and Johnson, M. N. (1974). Angiosarcoma of liver in the manufacture of polyvinyl chloride. *J. Occup. Environ. Med.* 16, 150-152.

[10] Angiosarcoma of the Liver Among Polyvinyl Chloride Workers -- Kentucky. [Online]. Available: https://www.cdc.gov/mmwr/preview/ mmwrhtml/lmrk103.htm. [Accessed: 30-Dec-2018].

[11] King, A. I., Viano, D. C., Mizeres, N., States, J. D. (1995). Humanitarian benefits of cadaver research on injury prevention. *J. Trauma* 38, 564–569.

[12] Death Certification: A Final Service to Your Patient — Chicago Medical Society. [Online]. Available: http://www.cmsdocs.org/news/ death-certification-a-final-service-to-your-patient. [Accessed: 27-Dec-2018].

[13] Ravakhah, K. (2006). Death certificates are not reliable: revivification of the autopsy. *South. Med. J.* 99, 728–733.

[14] Webber, B. J., Seguin, P. G., Burnett, D. G., Clark, L. L., Otto, J. L. (2012). Prevalence of and risk factors for autopsy-determined atherosclerosis among US service members, 2001-2011. *JAMA* 308, 2577–2583.

[15] Berenson, G. S., Srinivasan, S. R., Bao, W., Newman, W. P., Tracy, R. E., Wattigney, W. A. (1998). Association between multiple cardiovascular risk factors and atherosclerosis in children and young adults. The Bogalusa Heart Study. *N. Engl. J. Med.* 338, 1650–1656.

[16] U.S.D. of Justice (2016). Department of Justice report regarding the criminal investigation into the shooting death of Michael Brown by Ferguson, Missouri police officer Darren Wilson, CreateSpace Independent Publishing Platform.

[17] Nalli, N. R. (2018). Gunshot-wound dynamics model for John F. Kennedy assassination. *Heliyon* 4,

[18] Maeda, H., Ishikawa, T., Michiue, T. (2014). Forensic molecular pathology: Its impacts on routine work, education and training. *Leg. Med.* 16, 61–69.

[19] Hill, R. B. and Anderson, R. E. (1996). The recent history of the autopsy. *Arch. Pathol. Lab. Med.* 120, 702–712.

[20] Opsjøn, B. E. and Vogt, C. (2016). Explaining fetal death—what are the contributions of fetal autopsy and placenta examination? *Pediatr. Dev. Pathol.* 19, 24–30.

[21] Shojania, K. G., Burton, E. C., McDonald, K. M., Goldman, L. (2003). Changes in rates of autopsy-detected diagnostic errors over time: a systematic review. *JAMA* 289, 2849–2856.

[22] Pastores, S. M., Dulu, A., Voigt, L., Raoof, N., Alicea, M., Halpern, N. A. (2007). Premortem clinical diagnoses and postmortem autopsy findings: discrepancies in critically ill cancer patients. *Crit. Care Lond. Engl.* 11, R48.

[23] Winters, B., Custer, J., Galvagno, S. M., Colantuoni, E., Kapoor, S. G., Lee, H., et al. (2012). Diagnostic errors in the intensive care unit: a systematic review of autopsy studies. *BMJ Qual. Saf.* 21, 894–902.

[24] Mauf, S., Jentzsch, T., Laberke, P. J., Thali, M. J., Bartsch, C. (2016). Why we need postmortem analysis of cardiac implantable electronic devices. *J. Forensic Sci.* 61, 988–992.

[25] Ohrt-Nissen, S., Colville-Ebeling, B., Kandler, K., Hornbech, K., Steinmetz, J., Ravn, J., et al. (2016). Indication for resuscitative thoracotomy in thoracic injuries-adherence to the ATLS guidelines. A forensic autopsy based evaluation. *Injury* 47, 1019–1024.

[26] Joseph, B., Ibraheem, K., Haider, A. A., Kulvatunyou, N., Tang, A., O'Keefe, T., et al. (2016). Identifying potential utility of resuscitative endovascular balloon occlusion of the aorta: An autopsy study. *J. Trauma Acute Care Surg.* 81, S128–S132.

[27] Fraser, R. S. (1988). Lung perforation complicating tube thoracostomy: pathologic description of three cases. *Hum. Pathol.* 19, 518–523.

[28] Resnick, D. K. (1993). Delayed pulmonary perforation. A rare complication of tube thoracostomy. *Chest* 103, 311–313.

[29] Fitz, R. (1935). On perforating inflammation of the vermiform appendix with special reference to its early diagnosis and treatment. *N. Engl. J. Med.* 213, 245–248.

[30] Jahn, J. L., Giovannucci, E. L., Stampfer, M. J. (2015). The high prevalence of undiagnosed prostate cancer at autopsy: implications for epidemiology and treatment of prostate cancer in the prostate-specific antigen-era. *Int. J. Cancer J. Int. Cancer* 137, 2795–2802.

[31] Güth, U., Arndt, V., Stadlmann, S., Huang, D. J., Singer, G. (2015). Epidemiology in ovarian carcinoma: lessons from autopsy. *Gynecol. Oncol.* 138, 417–420.

[32] Ruangritchankul, K., Chindamporn, A., Worasilchai, N., Poumsuk, U., Keelawat, S., Bychkov, A. (2015). Invasive fungal disease in university hospital: a PCR-based study of autopsy cases. *Int. J. Clin. Exp. Pathol.* 8, 14840–14852.

[33] Chamilos, G., Luna, M., Lewis, R. E., Bodey, G. P., Chemaly, R., Tarrand, J. J., et al. (2006). Invasive fungal infections in patients with hematologic malignancies in a tertiary care cancer center: an autopsy study over a 15-year period (1989-2003). *Haematologica* 91, 986–989.

[34] Brosius, F. C., Waller, B. F., Roberts, W. C. (1981). Radiation heart disease. Analysis of 16 young (aged 15 to 33 years) necropsy patients who received over 3,500 rads to the heart. *Am. J. Med.* 70, 519–530.

[35] Veinot, J. P. and Edwards, W. D. (1996). Pathology of radiation-induced heart disease: a surgical and autopsy study of 27 cases. *Hum. Pathol.* 27, 766–773.

[36] Dong, J., Williams, N., Cerrone, M., Borck, C., Wand, D., Zhou, B., et al. (2018). Molecular autopsy: using the discovery of a novel de novo pathogenic variant in the KCNH2 gene to inform healthcare of surviving family. *Heliyon* 4, e01015.

[37] Tester, D. J., Medeiros-Domingo, A., Will, M. L., Haglund, C. M., Ackerman, M. J. (2012). Cardiac channel molecular autopsy: insights from 173 consecutive cases of autopsy-negative sudden unexplained death referred for postmortem genetic testing. *Mayo Clin. Proc.* 87, 524–539.

[38] Ackerman, M. J. (2009). State of postmortem genetic testing known as the cardiac channel molecular autopsy in the forensic evaluation of unexplained sudden cardiac death in the young. *Pacing Clin. Electrophysiol. PACE* 32 Suppl 2, S86-89.

[39] Sadler, T. W. (2011). *Langman's Medical Embryology*, Lippincott Williams & Wilkins.

[40] Chmielewski, P., Warchol, L., Gala-Błądzińska, A., Mróz, I., Walocha, J., Malczak, M., et al. (2016). Blood vessels of the shin - posterior tibial artery - anatomy - own studies and review of the literature. *Folia Med. Cracov.* 56, 5–9.

[41] McNamee, L. S., O'Brien, F. Y., Botha, J. H. (2009). Student perceptions of medico-legal autopsy demonstrations in a student-centred curriculum. *Med. Educ.* 43, 66–73.

[42] Burton, J. L. (2003). The autopsy in modern undergraduate medical education: a qualitative study of uses and curriculum considerations. *Med. Educ.* 37, 1073–1081.

[43] McPhee, S. J., Bottles, K., Lo, B., Saika, G., Crommie, D. (1986) .To redeem them from death. Reactions of family members to autopsy. *Am. J. Med.* 80, 665–671.

[44] Oppewal, F. and Meyboom-De Jong, B. (2001). Family members' experiences of autopsy. *Fam. Pract.* 18, 304–308.

[45] Rankin, J., Wright, C., Lind, T. (2002). Cross sectional survey of parents' experience and views of the postmortem examination. *BMJ* 324, 816–818.

In: A Closer Look at Autopsies
Editor: Fernando Robertson

ISBN: 978-1-53617-178-5
© 2020 Nova Science Publishers, Inc.

Chapter 7

RELIGIOUS PERSPECTIVES IN PERFORMING AUTOPSIES

*Lisa Kojima, Matthew Nagy
and Richard A. Prayson*, MD*

Cleveland Clinic Lerner College of Medicine
and Department of Anatomic Pathology, Cleveland, OH, US

ABSTRACT

Although religious beliefs about death and dying are variable, most religions believe autopsies are acceptable if desired by the individual and/or next of kin for special circumstances. Nonetheless, religion is a commonly cited reason for denying autopsy. The goal of this chapter is to examine religious beliefs around death and common reasons why religion may be invoked when deciding not to consent to an autopsy. Religions that will be examined include Judaism, Islam, Christianity (Catholicism and Protestantism), Christian Science, Church of Jesus Christ of Latter Day Saints (Mormon), Jehovah's Witness, Hinduism, and Buddhism.

* Corresponding Author's E-mail: praysor@ccf.org.

INTRODUCTION

Rates of autopsy in many developed countries, including the United States, have been declining since the latter half of the 20th century [1]. Although there is no single reason for this decline, religion is often cited as a major contributor, since family members will often invoke their religious beliefs to oppose autopsies [2]. Interestingly, however, none of the major world religions have doctrines that explicitly prohibit autopsies. In this chapter, we examine several different religions and their attitudes toward autopsies. It is important to note that views about autopsy not only vary between religions, but also within religious sects, depending on how individuals interpret their religious texts and teachings. Thus, we do not intend this to be an exhaustive summary, rather an attempt to provide context for practitioners working with religiously diverse patient populations.

JUDAISM

Judaism is the earliest of the Abrahamic religions (the others being Islam and Christianity), originally established around 1800 BCE. The central tenets of Judaism are contained in the Hebrew Bible (called the "Old Testament" in Christianity). The first five books of the Hebrew Bible is called the Torah, a collection of God's laws that were revealed to and recorded by Moses [3]. In addition to the Torah, Jewish law also stems from Jewish tradition and the Talmud, which is a collection of rabbinic teachings that are passed on from generation to generation. Together, the Torah, Talmud, and traditions make up the Jewish law termed *halacha* [4].

Within Judaism, there are three primary sects: Orthodox, Conservative, and Reformed. Those who practice Orthodox Judaism hold strictly to the laws of the Torah and the Talmud, whereas Reformed Jewish congregants reject many of the traditional beliefs of Orthodox Judaism [4]. Conservative Judaism was formed in response to the Reformed Jewish movement and constitutes a practice of Judaism that lies between the spectrum of Orthodox and Reformed Judaism [5]. Consequently, the stricter the sect, the more likely its members are to oppose autopsy on religious grounds [4].

Following death, the Torah commands that the body be buried on the same day of death [6]. There is an exception stated to this rule that the burial may be delayed in order to honor the dead, obtain a coffin, or to wait for either the family or the funeral orator [6]. Although autopsies are typically performed in the first 24 hours after death, even a prompt autopsy may prevent a quick burial. Some suggest if the autopsy was desired by the individual, honoring the wishes of the deceased may be an acceptable reason for delaying the burial [3].

There is also a command in the Torah against desecration of the dead, which is part and parcel of the belief that man is made in the image of God and thus deserves respect, even in death [7, 8]. As such, performing an autopsy would be a physical desecration of the body and may be deemed inappropriate. Some view delaying the burial or viewing the body as an act of desecration in and of itself [6]. Typically, the final authority on determining whether a specific autopsy would be considered a desecration is left to the judgement of a Rabbi [8].

While the above discusses some interpretations of *halacha* that may sway Jewish individuals away from autopsy, the issue is complicated by the Jewish principle, *pikuach nefesh. Pikuach nefesh* is a principle, established from the Torah and the Talmud, that suggests saving another's life is the greatest deed man can perform and takes precedence over most commandments (with exception to murder, adultery, and idol worship) [9]. The question of whether submission of one's body to an autopsy constitutes *pikuach nefesh* has been widely debated amongst Talmudic scholars for centuries. Some took the broad view that with so many diseases and medical conditions, autopsy is essential for the advancement of medical knowledge, and thus will eventually play a role in saving someone's life [6]. In this view, it would only be an act of desecration if the autopsy were performed for no reason [6]. Others say that abstract "medical advancements" do not qualify, but containing an epidemic or possibly uncovering a familial genetic disease would constitute saving a life [6]. Another subset of scholars argues that *pikuach nefesh* is only an acceptable justification to perform an autopsy if an immediate life will be saved, such as in the case of proving an accused murderer's innocence or rescuing an infant from a post-mortem mother's womb [3, 6].

When an autopsy is permitted, it is recommended that 1) it be performed as quickly as possible, 2) it be performed in a body bag to prevent loss of bodily fluid, 3) it be as non-intrusive as possible, 4) all organs be returned to their proper place or otherwise placed in a biodegradable bag, 5) all instruments be wiped clean and cloths placed in the body bag (as not to lose any blood), 6) genitalia and face be covered (if possible) out of modesty and respect, 7) and the body not be reopened, with incisions closed as tight as possible to prevent any body fluid from leaking out [4]. In some instances, a watchman may be asked to oversee the process to assure that procedures are accurately followed [4].

ISLAM

Islam, the world's second largest religion, has more than 1.5 billion followers worldwide, with the largest Muslim populations found in Asia, the Middle East, and Northern and Western Africa [10, 11, 12]. The two main branches of Islam—Sunni and Shi'ite—believe in one God, Allah, who is the creator and ruler of the universe [11, 13]. The Islamic law is called the Shari'a and is derived from the Islamic holy book called Qur'an and the Hadith, which include the words and deeds of the Prophet Mohammed, compiled after his death [11]. For issues that are not explicitly addressed in the Qur'an or the Hadith, reputable scholars will publish *fatawas* that lay out their opinion [10, 14, 15]. Since different scholars may hold different opinions, this may cause confusion for many Muslims [16].

In Islam, death is viewed as the will of Allah and a natural part of life [17]. Muslims will often oppose autopsies mainly based on three teachings found in the Shari'a. Because the Shari'a calls for Muslims to bury the dead as soon as possible, preferably within 24 hours, "in order to bring the dead person closer to what God has prepared for him/her," one of the main concerns for Muslims is that autopsies would delay the burial [3, 14]. Muslims also believe a prompt burial is essential in order for the body to not lose its human form [14]. Some have argued that a delay in burial is only allowed when more time is needed to properly prepare the body for burial [14]. The Shari'a also states that the deceased should be buried at or near the site of their death, preferably within 1 to 2 miles [3]. Transferring the deceased to a nearby hospital for an autopsy would prevent both of these from happening. Thirdly, Muslims believe that because the body belongs to Allah, the disfigurement of the body is forbidden and the sanctity of the body should not be violated [1, 14, 15, 17]. They will often quote the Prophet Muhammed, who said that "to break the bone of a dead person is like breaking the bone of a living person." Many have also interpreted this to mean that a deceased person can still experience pain [3, 15, 16].

Interestingly, however, autopsies are not directly addressed in the Qur'an or the Hadith [16]. Instead, several *fatawas* that were published during the 20th century may help inform Muslims regarding this topic [14]. In 1910, a *fatawa* was published called "Postmortem Examinations and the Postponement of Burial" [3, 14]. The scholar responsible for this *fatawa* stated that rushing to bury the person would risk the possibility that he or she may not be truly dead [14]. He applied this same reasoning to autopsies to claim that Muslims should view autopsies as beneficial and as a precautionary measure to avoid mistakes [14]. Regarding the issue of violating the sanctity of the body, Muslim scholars have pointed to the Islamic principle called *maslaha,* which states that if the benefits of the issue at hand outweighs the damages, then it should be allowed [3, 14]. A *fatawa* was published in 1952 in support of autopsies by invoking this idea of *maslaha* [3]. It explained that the Shari'a supports advances in medicine, and that a physician can only be fully educated when he understands the human anatomy not only from the outside but also from the inside. Thus, autopsies would be an instance in which "necessity allows what is prohibited" [18]. The Fatawa Committee at al-Azhar of 1982 also invoked *maslaha* to allow autopsies [3]. They claimed that if autopsies would allow medical students and doctors to increase their knowledge of the human body, would help control contagious diseases, or would serve justice, the benefits outweigh the negatives [16, 18].

After the *fatawas* were passed, Islam has allowed autopsies, particularly when the positives outweigh the negatives and when required by the law of the land [1, 10]. Nonetheless, autopsies remain unfavorable among Muslims. If they do consent, they will often request the autopsy to be performed with the utmost respect and that the funeral arrangements be made quickly [15].

CHRISTIANITY

Christianity, one of the three Abrahamic faiths, arose out of Judaism during the first century A. D. and quickly became a separate religion [19]. The word "Christianity" comes from the Hebrew word *Messiah*, or "The Anointed One," which Christians believe to be Jesus, the divine son of God [13]. Throughout the last two millennia, there have been disagreements over certain doctrines, which resulted in many different churches and denominations. The Roman Catholic Church is the single largest Christian church in the world, with over a billion followers [13]. The other main branch of Christianity is referred to as Protestantism, which includes the Anglican Communion and the Free Churches, the latter of which encompasses churches that arose in the United States and do not conform to the Roman Catholic or the Anglican Communion traditions [13]. Despite debates regarding certain doctrinal issues, all forms of Christianity agree that there is only one God, who reveals himself in the Trinity as the Father, the Son (Jesus), and the Holy Spirit [13].

There are no Christian laws or edicts that forbid autopsies, although the dignity of the deceased person must be respected [16, 20]. There is much historical evidence highlighting the church's support for autopsy [2]. The Pope of the Roman Catholic Church has historically allowed and even encouraged dissections. For example, in 1209, Pope Innocent III issued a statement recommending that experienced physicians evaluate the bodies of people whose deaths were unexplained [21]. Prior to this, the church was against violating the bodies, but Pope Innocent III's statement marked a reversal in this thought [21]. During the Middle Ages when the plague killed many Europeans, the Pope required autopsies to be performed to find a cause of the plague [16]. During the 15th century, Pope Sixtus IV issued a bull, which was later confirmed by Pope Clement VII, allowing medical students in Bologna and Padua to dissect and study human bodies [2, 22, 23]. Throughout the Renaissance era, the church often allowed artists, such as Leonardo da Vinci to perform dissections to better understand the human anatomy [16]. More recently, during the 20th century, Pope Pius XII claimed that autopsies are acceptable as long as the body is treated with respect and the family has provided consent to the procedure [22].

Despite precedents in support of autopsies, the perception that the Catholic Church opposes autopsies still developed, for which there may be a historical basis. During the 13th century, the bodies of Crusaders who died in the Holy Land were cut up and boiled so that their remains could be taken home for a proper burial [2]. The pope at the time, Pope Boniface VII, described these practices as inhuman and barbaric, and ruled against them. Although this affected anatomists who boiled the bodies to prepare the bones for their studies, it was not intended to prevent anatomic studies using dissections. In fact, public dissections began in 1302, only two years after the pope's ruling, at a papal university called University of Bologna. Despite the papal support for dissections, misinformation surrounding this time period may have contributed to the negative perception of autopsies.

The Protestant church also supports autopsies based on the belief that they provide one last opportunity for the person to serve God and contribute to humanity [20, 24]. Historically, however, there were mostly negative attitudes toward autopsies in Protestant countries [20]. Before the first English anatomic law was passed at the end of the 19th century, executed criminals were often used for anatomic dissections and studies [2, 20]. In addition, because autopsies were not widely accepted in countries under Protestant rule and there was a limited number of bodies available, autopsies became associated with grave-robbing [2, 20]. As a result, people often associated autopsies with crime and developed negative opinions of autopsies [20].

In conclusion, Christianity does not have any religious prohibitions on autopsy, although individual members of the clergy may advise against consenting [1, 16]. Additionally, because of certain historical events, as well as potential misinformation of these events, Christians may be reluctant to consent to autopsies [2].

CHRISTIAN SCIENCE

The Mother Church of the Christian Science religion was founded by Mary Baker Eddy in 1879 in Massachusetts. Eddy established this church in response to a miraculous healing she received when reading about the healings of Jesus in the Bible [25]. She also published the book "Science and Health with Key to the Scriptures," or just "Science and Health," in 1875 which is upheld as the full explanation for the biblical foundation on which one can receive spiritual regeneration and healing [25, 26]. In order to better understand reasons in which Christian Scientists may object to autopsy, it is important to provide a brief overview of the relationship between the Mother Church and the medical community.

While Christian Scientists admit to and acknowledge the physical nature of illness, they argue that the origin of illness is not rooted in a condition of the physical, but rather in the metaphysical realm of the heart [26]. Rather than medicine itself being a cure, they believe medicine will provide only transient relief and that proper communion with God is the only way to bring true healing. As such, certain members of the church are trained as Christian Science practitioners to offer support via prayer in order to facilitate healing [27]. While Christian Scientist congregants have the right to utilize medical services, many will forego modern medical treatment, as it is believed that the two are incompatible with each other [26, 27].

In this context, there is general reluctance to participate in the practice of autopsy as contributing to the advancement of medical knowledge and treatment would be seen to be of no benefit. As such, autopsy is not typically accepted in Christian Science, except in the case of sudden death or when required by law [20, 26]. When autopsy is permitted, it is preferred that the body of a female be prepared by another female [26]. The reason in which autopsy is permitted in the case of sudden death is not explicitly stated, but there is evidence both from Eddy's writings and life. In "Science and Health," Eddy writes of an instance where a woman died after being forcibly anesthetized for a surgery. An autopsy was then performed which led to a court ruling that the death was caused by the fear induced by the physicians [28]. In a more personal instance, following the death of Eddy's husband, an autopsy was performed to determine cause of death. Despite the discovery of defects in his heart valves, Eddy claimed that the autopsy revealed her husband was killed by a mental assassination [25, 29]. As such, both cases allow for the use of autopsy to substantiate the claims of the role of the metaphysical, rather than physical, in precipitating death.

CHURCH OF JESUS CHRIST OF LATTER DAY SAINTS (MORMON)

The Church of Jesus Christ of Latter Day Saints (LDS) was established by Joseph Smith in 1830 [30]. In his youth, Smith received a vision from God the Father and Jesus Christ, who taught him that the churches of his time were steeped in sin and failed to follow His commandments. It was not until years later that he would receive a vision from an angel, which would ultimately lead him to discover golden plates buried on a hill that contained a previously undiscovered testament of Jesus Christ, the Book of Mormon [31]. This book was not to replace, but supplement the Holy Bible of the Christian faith to restore the church, which eventually became the Church of Jesus Christ of Latter Day Saints [31]. The church claims to be unique as its leadership has continued to receive and record instances of divine revelations, such is recorded in two additional texts that have become standard works of the church, "Doctrines and Covenants" and the

"Pearl of Great Price." Members of the church are often referred to as Mormons, but prefer the title Latter Day Saints [32].

The Latter Day Saints believe every person exists eternally both before birth and after death [3]. During earthly life, both the body and spirit are essential in exaltation, and thus the two are intimately intertwined [30]. As such, Latter Day Saints are encouraged to utilize the prevention and treatment of disease offered by modern medicine, as they hold that both science and faith play important roles in healing. In general, church leadership does not condone the practice of trusting in either extreme: faith healing only versus a science only approach [33].

In regard to autopsy, there is no community stance on the issue, rather it is permitted if it is the family's decision or if it is necessary to comply with the law. This likely stems from the belief that after death, the spirit leaves the body and returns home to God. When the resurrection occurs, all who have passed will receive a new body, but this will be a spiritual body separate from the body on earth [33]. As such, the General Handbook of Instruction, which is the official manual for church policy and practice, notes autopsy as a "medical" rather than a "moral" consideration [34]. Moreover, it is stated in the Encyclopedia of Mormonism that by utilizing autopsy as a method to determine cause of death and train future health care providers, "both those who die and those who examine them contribute to improving the quality of life and health of their fellow human beings" [35].

JEHOVAH'S WITNESS

The Jehovah's Witnesses were established in the late 1800's by Charles Taze Russell and a small Bible study group, when they began publishing a magazine called "Zions Watchtower and Herald of Christ's Presence" [36]. Jehovah's Witnesses hold the Holy Bible as inerrant, as do most Christian faiths, but diverge in the belief that Jehova (God) is still revealing new truths about his kingdom [37]. Additionally, Jehovah's Witnesses believe Jesus is both the Son of God and the Messiah, though they do not believe that he himself is God, but that there is one God, Jehova [38, 39]. Interpretations of the Bible and current events are communicated in their bi-monthly publications, "The Watchtower" and "Awake!" [40].

Jehovah's Witnesses are most famously known in the health care world for rejecting the use of blood products in their medical care. Abstaining from blood transfusion stems from their interpretation of biblical passages which instruct one not to ingest blood [41]. Refusing blood treatment is also a testament of respect to God as the giver of life, as blood is viewed as being a representation of life [41]. This issue is very important to Jehovah's Witnesses, as the consequences of transgressing this command unrepentantly could result in severing one's relationship with God and forfeiting eternal life [36, 42].

Despite the prohibition against blood transfusion, the Jehovah's Witness community does not have strong opinions about autopsy, particularly because it is not mentioned in the Bible and death is interpreted as a state of pure nothingness [3]. The exception to this could be apprehension from a family that blood may be improperly handled or taken from the cadaver [36]. Interestingly, autopsy is explicitly mentioned three times in the official magazine "Awake!," yet it is only discussed as a matter of fact rather than debate [43, 44, 45]. If autopsy is required by the law, Witnesses will typically agree in concordance with the biblical command to "let every soul be in subjection to the superior authorities" [46].

HINDUISM

Hinduism has particularly old origins, dating back as early as 2500 BCE, and is observed more as a philosophy rather than a religion [13]. There is no specific text that defines orthodoxy, though classical Hinduism was formed through the interaction of Vedic traditions, Buddhism, and Jainism. As such, diverse beliefs exist within Hinduism due to the lack of doctrinal restraints [47]. There are approximately one billion Hindus in the world, with the majority residing in India and over a million living in the United States [13].

Despite the diversity in Hindu beliefs, most believe in reincarnation, which suggests each living being has had multiple existences in the past and will have more in the future [47]. Thus, the life one currently lives is determined by quality of their past life, and their fate following death will be determined by their present life, also known as Karma [48]. As such, it is possible to improve with each successive life, but the ultimate goal is to be free from the cycle of birth and rebirth. The only way to escape this cycle is by reaching enlightenment with the ultimate reality, known as the brahman. Many believe that enlightenment may be reached when one has lived a virtuous life and died a "good" death [48].

A "good" death is said to occur when the final thought of one's life is focused on the brahman [48]. Following death, the tradition is for the body to be cremated (usually within 24 hours) and for the ashes to be spread out over holy water, in order to purify that which is now impure [49]. As such, delaying cremation for an autopsy may be grounds for a Hindu family to deny post-mortem examination [50]. Additionally, mourning by the family is common both leading up to the death and afterwards, which may leave the family in a position to be less open to autopsy as an option [47]. Furthermore, although the soul is believed to leave the body following death, it remains aware. Thus, performing an autopsy on the body, rather than providing the last rites of cremation, may hurt or disturb the soul of the deceased [49]. If the law requires autopsy, most will agree, though it may be requested that the deceased 1) not be touched by non-Hindus (unless wearing gloves), 2) be wrapped in white cloth, and 3) that jewelry and other religious or sacred items be left on the body [13].

BUDDHISM

Buddhism, one of the three Dharmic faiths, has more than 700 million followers in East Asia and South East Asia [13]. It was founded by a Hindu Prince, Siddhartha Gautama, during the sixth century BCE [13],

[19]. There are three schools of thought within Buddhism: Mahayana, Tibetan, and Theravada [13, 19]. As a religion that stemmed out of Hinduism, Buddhism shares similar beliefs such as reincarnation. However, unlike Hinduism, Buddhism does not believe in the caste system, a god, or divine judgement [13]. Buddhism does not have any religious prohibition on autopsy, given the belief that it would be a way of serving others, an essential principle in Buddhism [1]. Autopsies are permitted after the deceased's soul has made its transition, which is three days after death or earlier, as determined by a Buddhist teacher [20]. There are no official Buddhist rituals after death, although a monk or minister from the same school should be notified promptly [13].

CONCLUSION

Physicians will undoubtedly continue to encounter patients who deny autopsies on the basis of their religious beliefs. While none of the major religions have an explicit ban on autopsy, varying interpretations of texts and historical events may nonetheless result in denial of autopsy. As the United States becomes increasingly diverse, it is important for practitioners to understand the context from which these oppositions may stem, in order to be sensitive and compassionate toward patients and their families.

REFERENCES

[1]   Burton, J. L. and Underwood, J. (2007). Clinical, Educational, and Epidemiological Value of Autopsy. *The Lancet*, 369(9571): 1471–80.

[2]   Geller, S. A. (1984). Religious Attitudes and the Autopsy. *Archives of Pathology & Laboratory Medicine*, 108(6): 494–96.

[3]   Burton, E. C. and Beal, S. "Religions and the Autopsy." *Medscape.* https://emedicine.medscape.com/article/1705993-overview#a2 (Accessed January 19, 2019).

[4]   Goodman, N. R., Goodman, J. L. and Hofman, W.I. (2011). Autopsy: Traditional Jewish Laws and Customs 'Halacha.' *The American Journal of Forensic Medicine and Pathology*, 32(3): 300–303.

[5]   Karp, A. J. (1986). A Century of Conservative Judaism in the United States. *The American Jewish Year Book*, 86: 3–61.

[6]   Misher, J. "Autopsies in Jewish Law: A Dissection of the Sources." *YUTorah Online*. https://www.yutorah.org/lectures/lecture.cfm/ 799112/jason-misher/autopsies-in-jewish-law-a-dissection-of-the-sources/ (Accessed January 19, 2019).

[7]   Kwaghe, B. V., Manasseh, A. N., Elachi, U. G., Emmmanuel, I., Silas, O. A., Titus, N. F., Akpa, P. O., Jimoh, A. A. and Mandong, B. M. (2017). Autopsy and the Religious Beliefs of Christians, Muslims and Jews: a Short Review of the Historical Perspective. *Jos Journal of Medicine*, 11(2): 62–64.

[8]   Lamm, M. *The Jewish Way in Death and Mourning*. Middle Village, NY: Jonathan David Publishers, 2000.

[9]   Eisenberg, R. L. "Death." In *The JPS Guide to Jewish Traditions*, 1st ed. Philadelphia: The Jewish Publication Society, 2004. 74–124.

[10] Mohammed, M. and Kharoshah, M. A. (2014). Autopsy in Islam and Current Practice in Arab Muslim Countries. *Journal of Forensic and Legal Medicine*, 23: 80–83.

[11] Inhorn, M. C. and Serour, G. I. (2011). Islam, Medicine, and Arab-Muslim Refugee Health in America after 9/11. *The Lancet*, 378(9794): 935–43.

[12] *Mapping the Global Muslim Population*. Pew Research Center. http://www.pewforum.org/2009/10/07/mapping-the-global-muslim-population/ (Accessed January 19, 2019).

[13] Burton, J. L., and Rutty, G. "Religious Attitudes to Death and Post-Mortem Examinations." In *The Hospital Autopsy: A Manual of Fundamental Autopsy Practice*. 3rd ed. London: Hodder Arnold, 2010. 39-58.

[14] Rispler-Chaim, V. (1993). The Ethics of Postmortem Examinations in Contemporary Islam. *Journal of Medical Ethics*, 19(3): 164–68.

[15] Sajid, M. I. (2016). Autopsy in Islam: Considerations for Deceased Muslims and Their Families Currently and in the Future. *The American Journal of Forensic Medicine and Pathology*, 37(1): 29–31.

[16] Davis, G. J. and Peterson, B. R. (1996). Dilemmas and Solutions for the Pathologist and Clinician Encountering Religious Views of the Autopsy. *Southern Medical Journal*, 89(11): 1041–44.

[17] Chichester, M. (2007). Requesting Perinatal Autopsy: Multicultural Considerations. *The American Journal of Maternal/Child Nursing*, 32(2): 81.

[18] Al-Adnani, M. and Scheimberg, I. (2006). How Can We Improve the Rate of Autopsies among Muslims? *British Medical Journal*, 332(7536): 310.

[19] Rutty, J. E. "Religious Attitudes to Death: What Every Pathologist Needs to Know." In *Essentials of Autopsy Practice*. Vol. 1. London: Springer, 2001. 1-22.

[20] Connolly, A. J., Finkbeiner, W. E., Ursell, P. C. and Davis, R. L. "Legal, Social, and Ethical Issues." In *Autopsy Pathology: A Manual and Atlas*. 3rd ed. Philadelphia: Elsevier, 2016. 15–23.

[21] Campos, F. P. F and Rocha, L. O. S. (2015). The Pedagogical Value of Autopsy. *Autopsy & Case Reports*, 5(3): 1–6.

[22] Gordijn, S. J., Erwich, J. J. and Khong, T. Y. (2007). The Perinatal Autopsy: Pertinent Issues in Multicultural Western Europe. *European Journal of Obstetrics & Gynecology and Reproductive Biology*, 132(1): 3–7.

[23] Dada, M. A. and Ansari, N. A. (1996). Origins of the Postmortem Examination in Diagnosis. *Journal of Clinical Pathology*, 49(12): 965–66.

[24] Boglioli, L. R. and Taff, M. L. (1990). Religious Objection to Autopsy: An Ethical Dilemma for Medical Examiners. *Journal of Forensic Medicine*, 11(1): 1–8.

[25] Gottschalk, S. *The Emergence of Christian Science in American Religious Life*. Berkeley, CA: University of California Press, 1978.

[26] Abbott, D. *The Christian Science Tradition: Religious Beliefs and Healthcare Decisions.* Chicago: Park Ridge Center for the Study of Health, Faith, and Ethics, 2002.

[27] Gazelle, G., Glover, C. and Stricklin, S. L. (2004). Care of the Christian Science Patient. *Journal of Palliative Medicine*, 7(4): 585–88.

[28] Eddy, M. B. "Chapter VI: Science, Theology, and Medicine." In *Science and Health with Key to the Scriptures.* Boston, MA: The Christian Science Board of Directors, 1875.

[29] Georgine, M. *The Life of Mary Baker G. Eddy: And the History of Christian Science.* 1909. Reprint, Miami, FL: HardPress Publishing, 2013.

[30] Simmerman, S. R. (1993). The Mormon Health Traditions: An Evolving View of Modern Medicine. *Journal of Religion and Health*, 32(3): 189–96.

[31] *Saints: The Story of the Church of Jesus Christ in the Latter Days, Vol. 1.* Salt Lake City, UT: The Church of Jesus Christ of Latter-day Saints, 2018.

[32] Manscill, C. K. "The Explanatory Introduction: A Guide to the Doctrine and Covenants." In *Sperry Symposium Classics: The Doctrine and Covenants.* Provo, UT: Religious Studies Center, Brigham Young University, 2004. 56–67.

[33] Abbott, D. *The Latter-Day Saints Tradition: Religious Beliefs and Healthcare Decisions.* Chicago: Park Ridge Center for the Study of Health, Faith, and Ethics, 2002.

[34] Allan, F. D. *Encyclopedia of Mormonism.* "Autopsy." New York: Macmillan Publishing Company, 1992.

[35] "Handbook 2: Administering the Church." Salt Lake City, UT: The Church of Jesus Christ of Latter-day Saints, 2018.

[36] DuBose, E. R. *The Jehovah's Witness Tradition: Religious Beliefs and Healthcare Decisions.* Chicago: Park Ridge Center for the Study of Health, Faith, and Ethics, 2002.

[37] "Jehovah, the God of Progressive Revelation." *The Watchtower,* June 15, 1964. https://wol.jw.org/en/wol/d/r1/lp-e/1964442 (Accessed January 19, 2019).

[38] "Jesus Christ—God's Beloved Son." *The Watchtower,* June 1, 1988. https://wol.jw.org/en/wol/d/r1/lp-e/1988403 (Accessed January 19, 2019).

[39] "Is the Trinity a Bible Teaching?" *The Watchtower*, March 1, 2012. https://www.jw.org/en/publications/magazines/wp20120301/Is-the-Trinity-a-Bible-teaching/ (Accessed January 19, 2019).

[40] Wah, C. R. (2001). An Introduction to Research and Analysis of Jehovah's Witnesses: A View from the Watchtower. *Review of Religious Research*, 43(2): 161–74.

[41] "The Real Value of Blood." *Awake!*, August 2006. https://www.jw.org/en/publications/magazines/g200608/The-Real-Value-of-Blood/ (Accessed January 19, 2019).

[42] Muramoto, O. (2001). Bioethical Aspects of the Recent Changes in the Policy of Refusal of Blood by Jehovah's Witnesses. *British Medical Journal*, 322(7277): 37–39.

[43] "Modern Medicine—How High Can It Reach?" *Awake!*, June 8, 2001. https://www.jw.org/en/publications/magazines/g20010608/Modern-Medicine-How-High-Can-It-Reach/ (Accessed January 19, 2019).

[44] "Ignaz Semmelweis." *Awake!*, November 3, 2016. https://www.jw.org/en/publications/magazines/awake-no3-2016-june/ignaz-semmelweis-childbed-fever-germ-theory/ (Accessed January 19, 2019).

[45] "I Accepted God's View of Blood." *Awake!*, December 8, 2003. https://www.jw.org/en/publications/magazines/g20031208/I-Accepted-Gods-View-of-Blood/ (Accessed January 19, 2019).

[46] "Christian Obedience to Law." In *The Truth That Leads to Eternal Life*. The Watchtower, 1981. 157–62.

[47] Sharma, A. *The Hindu Tradition: Religious Beliefs and Healthcare Decisions*. Chicago: Park Ridge Center for the Study of Health, Faith, and Ethics, 2002.

[48] Firth, S. (2005). End-of-Life: A Hindu View. *The Lancet*, 366(9486): 682–86.

[49] *What Is Hinduism? Modern Adventures into a Profound Global Faith*. 1st ed. Kapaa, Hawaii: Himalayan Academy, 2007.

[50] Rudra, A. and Murty, O. P. (2014). Attitude to Organ Donation and Autopsy in Different Religious Denominations. *Journal of Forensic Medicine and Toxicology*, 31(2): 54–56.

INDEX

ADVANCES IN THERAPEUTICS AND DIAGNOSTICS OF HUMAN DISEASES

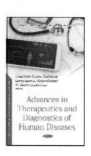

EDITORS: S. Gowtham Kumar, Langeswaran Kulathaivel, and N. Madhusudhanan

SERIES: Medical Procedures, Testing and Technology

BOOK DESCRIPTION: This reference book equips readers with cutting-edge information on the many advances in diagnostic and therapeutic treatments for human diseases that have been made in recent years, with examples from laboratory medicine.

HARDCOVER ISBN: 978-1-53615-382-8
RETAIL PRICE: $230

PROGRESS IN MEDICAL RESEARCH: GOVERNMENT PROGRAMS AND KEY ISSUES

EDITOR: Nima Gustavsson

SERIES: Medical Procedures, Testing and Technology

BOOK DESCRIPTION: During the 115th Congress, several bipartisan bills were introduced that aimed to expand the number of telehealth services that are covered under Medicare. Telehealth is the electronic delivery of a health care service via a technological method.

SOFTCOVER ISBN: 978-1-53614-105-4
RETAIL PRICE: $82

To see a complete list of Nova publications, please visit our website at www.novapublishers.com

Related Nova Publications

ELISA: HISTORY, TYPES AND APPLICATIONS

EDITOR: Md Rezaul Karim

SERIES: Medical Procedures, Testing and Technology

BOOK DESCRIPTION: *ELISA: History, Types and Applications* contains unique combinations of chapters in which the abstract of each chapter defines the work considered for the entire chapter. One of the essential goals of this book is to delineate vital information about different types of ELISA and their applications.

HARDCOVER ISBN: 978-1-53614-393-5
RETAIL PRICE: $160

To see a complete list of Nova publications, please visit our website at www.novapublishers.com